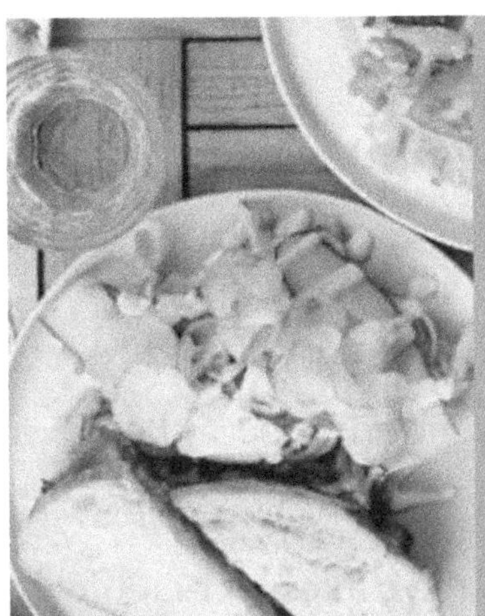

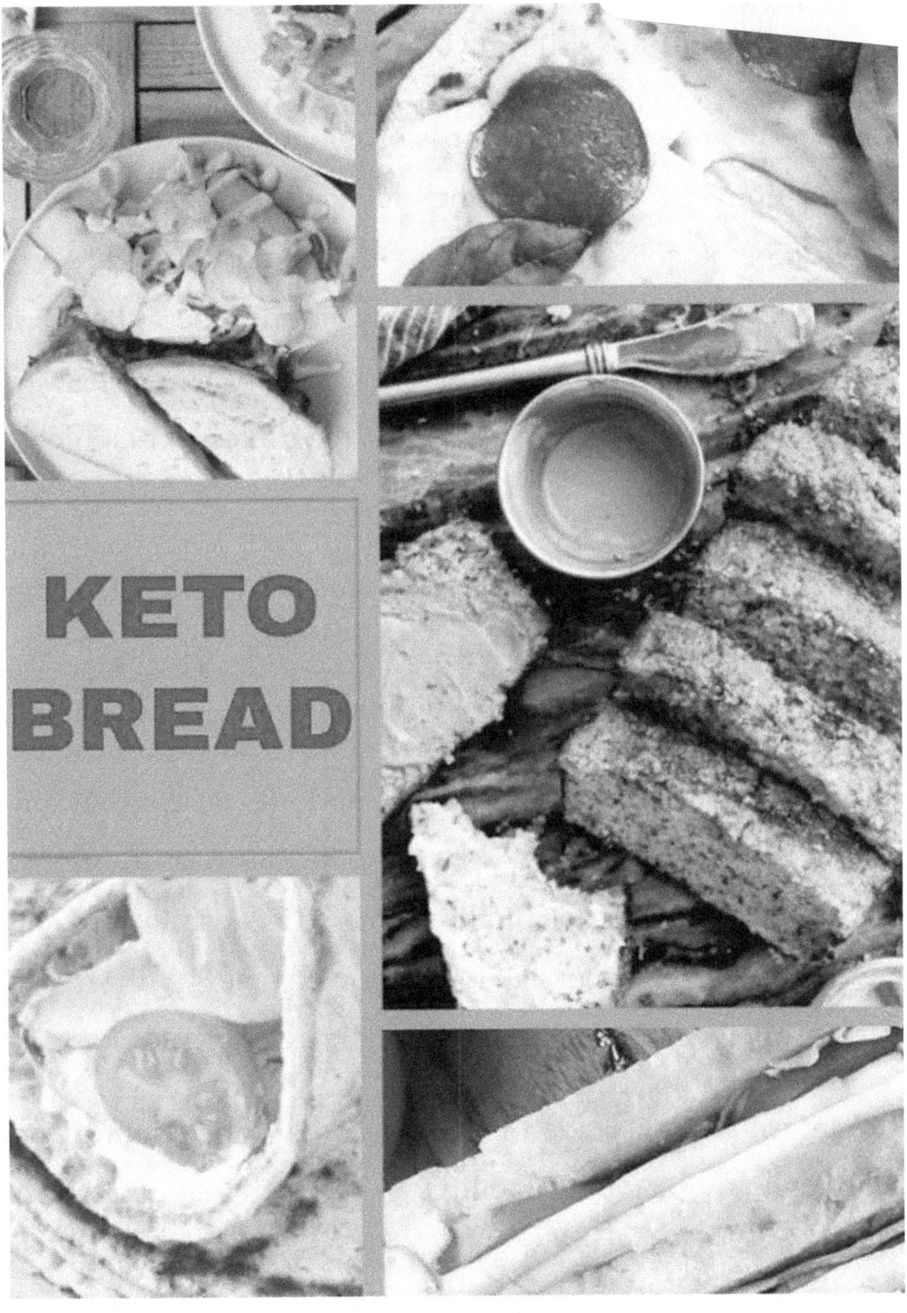

KETO
BREAD

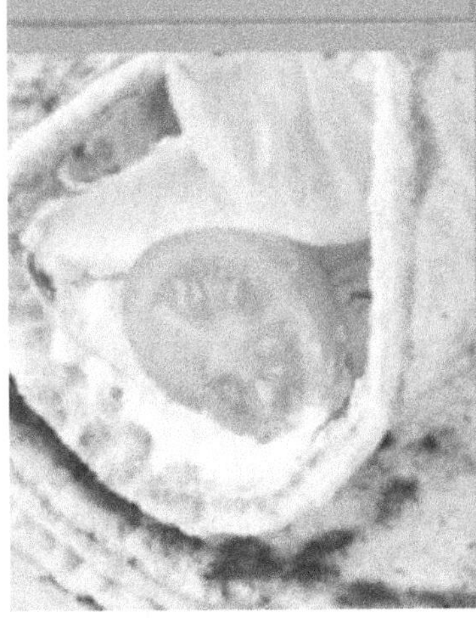

Table Of Contents

INTRODUCTION

Bread is satisfying and nutritious food items; however, not all bread is the same when it comes to their nutritive value. Some types of bread are typically lower in carbohydrate content; this makes them higher in protein, iron, fiber, and several other minerals. Bread made from whole grains and whole wheat is low carb bread. They contain protein-rich ingredients such as lentils, flaxseed, and oats.

Low carb bread is ideal for people who are trying to lose a few inches of body fat. Carbohydrates contain extra calories; hence, those who have a sedentary lifestyle fail to use up the calories that end up staying inside the body. Moreover, some people need to control or stabilize their blood sugar because of diabetes. Bread low in carb is also low in sugar content; thus making the bread perfect for this medical condition.

Choose the kind of bread that you eat to make sure that you receive low contents of carbohydrate. Whole wheat bread and tortillas are generally lower in carb. In fact, any bread made from barley, oats, soy flour and wheat gluten qualify as low carb bread. More gluten content in bread makes them lower in carbohydrates and higher in protein. For instance, a small piece of tortilla made from gluten has about 11 grams of carbohydrates; this is much lower, as compared to the 25 grams in regular tortillas.

Aside from adding more gluten, sprouting is another way to reduce the number of carbohydrates in bread. Sprouted grain bread is flourless; it merely contains lentils, oats, barley, and soy. Although sprouting may take several days, it is worth the effort because of its nutritive value and health benefits. Milling the flour, as done in making white flour, removes the bran and germ of the kernels. Hence, bread made from this flour is lower in protein and higher in carbohydrates. Hence, sprouted grains are definitely a healthier option than refined grains.

You will surely enjoy the taste of low carb bread, particularly if you add in ingredients that would give it a delightful taste. Opt for this type of bread that is tasty, low in calories and high in protein and other essential vitamins and minerals.

In this eBook, you will find everything you need to know about keto bread, how they can benefit the body and the truth about low carb, you will find out if cutting carbs from your diet will help you lose weight, healthy high fat recipes, easy keto recipes and recipes for beginners.

UNDERSTANDING WHAT LOW CARB DIET IS

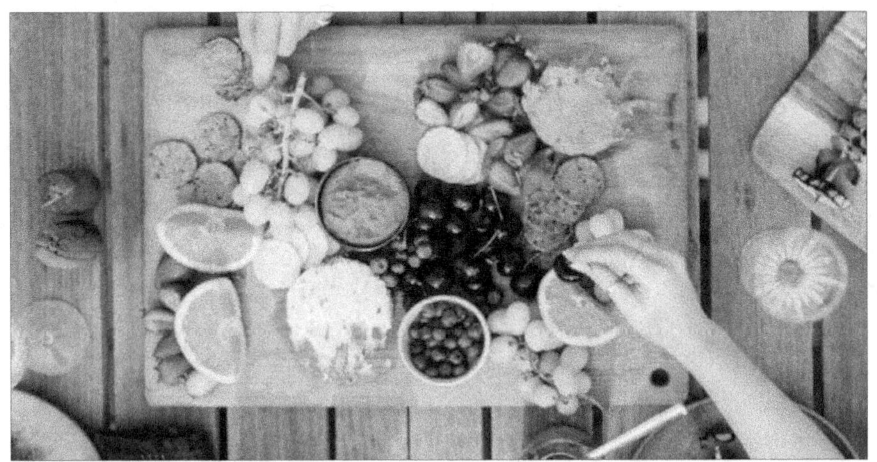

When planning to lose weight, there is usually some type of eating regimen, which must be observed. These diets are necessarily included to complement the exercise program, you engage in. Normally these plans mainly consist of foods that are low in carbohydrates. This is consistent with your weight loss goals. Therefore, a popular diet program for many fitness buffs is a low carb diet.

Weight gain often occurs when your intake of calorie-rich foods are not sufficiently burned. Obviously, still, some kind of burning takes place inside your body. Unfortunately, this combustion is not done at a level where you can lose significant weight.

When you exercise, the body is pushed to burn fat and sugar at a faster pace. Thus, significant weight loss or otherwise obtained in this case.

The problem is that after participating in strenuous physical activities, exercises will naturally feel hunger pangs, a need that they must meet. If they have no effective and healthy eating program, a goal of losing physical weight, will not be reached.

With a low carb diet, but your training routines are effectively complemented. Therefore, weight loss ceases to be an elusive goal.

With this particular diet program, there is often a piece of very specific meal information included that will serve as your guide when trying to lose weight. Specifically, this information may be found in the number of food servings are allowed, how many calories are contained in each diet foods and diet drinks, the weight of your diet food (presented in grams or ounces), and the quantity of food, beverages, as you are allowed to consume.

At first glance, this list above may seem too strict. However, if you are serious about losing weight, you will find this information and the low carb diet quite effective. This is because, apart from physical training offered by your training program, this diet plan also trains your body to follow a specific and healthy eating habit. Ultimately, you are able to fully enjoy your weight loss program.

Just a quick and final reminder. A typical low carb diet will usually include the ingestion of lowfat drink. Low fat means little if no sugar. In this context, fruit juices such as oranges often a highly recommended beverage type of dieting individuals. But when an option involving an orange and its juice form, the latter carries more calories. Therefore, if you plan to consume fruits as a part of your diet, it is always recommended that you take them in solid form.

BASICS FOR STARTING
A LOW CARB DIET

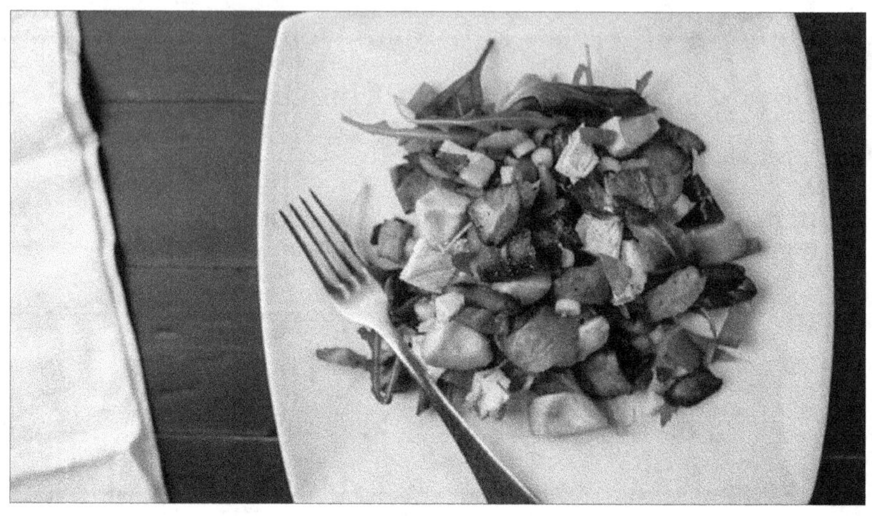

Low carb diets have become popular because they are an easy way to lose weight fast.

Before starting on a low carb eating plan, educate yourself on the types of foods you can eat. It is also helpful to have a quick reference guide for counting the grams of carbs in various foods. In the beginning stages of the diet, you will want to limit your daily net carb count at about 30 grams. Net carbs are the total carbs minus the fiber. The daily carb intake varies so you will need to determine the best level for you to continue losing weight. The key is to eat fewer carbohydrates than your body burns in a day. Typically, the carbs can be slowly increased as long as weight loss continues. People with slower metabolisms will need to keep the carb count extremely low for the duration of the diet in order to continue to lose weight. Taking a supplement to boost metabolism or consulting a doctor regarding prescription medications may be required if ongoing weight loss becomes difficult.

Preparing your own meals is less costly than buying prepared foods and it is easier to keep track of the carb counts. The internet is full of free low carb recipes and there are a number of good low carb cookbooks. Learn the basics of low carb cooking and the types of ingredients used. Almond meal and coconut flour are excellent substitutes for flour. Both natural and artificial sweeteners are available to replace sugar in dessert recipes. Having a good collection of recipes on hand will get you off to a good start when planning meals.

Now is a good time to go through the food in your kitchen to get rid of anything that may be a temptation. Items that contain flour and/or sugar should be eliminated. If other family members insist on having high carb foods around, you will need to come up with a plan to stay away from them. The good news is that there are delicious low carb substitutes to replace these forbidden foods. Having plenty of great tasting low carb foods around will prevent the urge to eat sugary snacks.

You will need to read food labels while shopping. A good rule of thumb is to stick with foods that are less than 10 net grams of carbs per serving. While in the grocery store, your shopping should be focused on the perimeter of the store. The aisles are loaded with processed foods that are usually high in carbs. The primary low carb staples are protein-rich foods such as eggs, cheese, and meat. It's also important to eat plenty of low carb fruits and vegetables. Use a carbcounting reference guide to determine which foods to choose. Low carb protein bars, sugar-free ice cream, nuts and cheese sticks are popular snacks. Sugar-free candies are readily available, but be aware that many are made with sugar alcohols which can cause stomach distress.

Transitioning to a lower carb diet may seem difficult at first, but remember things will get easier. Eating small portions every couple of hours is better than waiting 5 hours or more for meal times. There is no need to worry about the amount of food as long as the net carbs are within reason. Be sure to drink plenty of water as it is helpful to keep the body flushing out wastes. Weigh yourself every few days to make sure you are continuing to lose weight. Adjust your daily net carb intake as needed to stay on track.

EASY LOW CARB DIET - YOUR QICK GUIDE

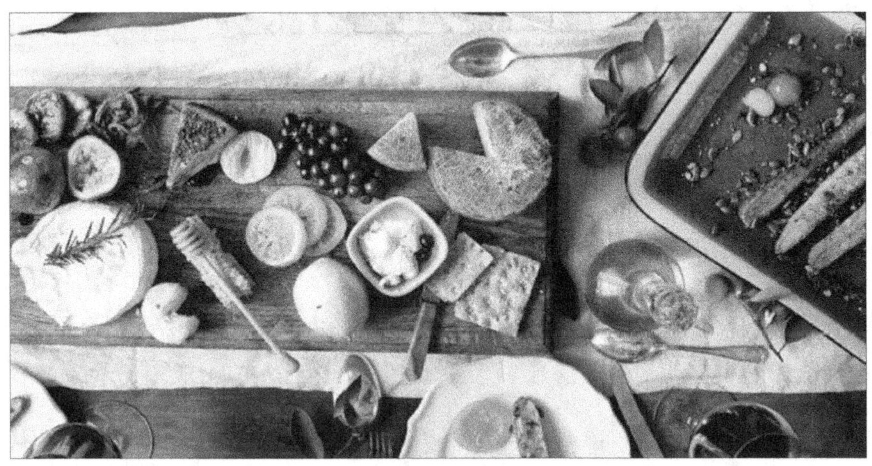

It is surprising why most people think that there is no such thing as an easy low carb diet. These people can't be blamed because let's face it - we are not talking about only a few pounds here. As a matter of fact, 31% of the world's total population is considered overweight and 10% is considered obese. Because of these, different diet methods are all over the place and one of these is the low carb diet, but then again, there are many low carb diet methods all over the place, and the reason why you've come across this ebook is because you were searching for an easy low carb diet that could help you shed those extra pounds easily. Well, congratulations because this article aims to provide you an ultimate and quick guide on the real concept of low carbohydrate diet and what it can actually do for you.

What are low carbohydrate diets? Low carb diets mainly focus on the utilization of energy as well as the controlling energy levels acquired and released from carbs, which are the body's primary energy source. The main objective of a low carbohydrate diet is to stimulate the body to start utilizing fat as its main source of energy instead of the carbohydrates. The concept is simple; thus, there is such a thing as an easy low carb diet. Now, if you have already decided to take the low carb diet, what's next? Well, it's high time to start thinking ahead so that you can start enjoying your weight loss success. Read on and learn from this easy low carb diet quick guide.

1. Become informed

Anything is easier when you are equipped with enough information. Before embarking into the low carbohydrate diet, it is a good idea to read books about it and familiarize yourself with the concepts and principles. Above all, never ever fall for the myths of eating low carbs.

2. Be prepared for making easy changes

Easy low carb diet starts with easy changes. Easy changes mean making gradual changes to your habits until finally get over with the bad old habits. You can do this easily by changing one or two things at a time. You will surely be surprised with how much you can achieve with less and easier effort than you ever thought.

3. Familiarize yourself with what you can eat

Most of us think more about what we can't eat; however, we can be more productive and successful when we think of the foods that we can eat. At first, you've got to make it simple, for instance, you can still eat the same lunch except that you've got to eat vegetables instead of starch.

4. Make plans for the first week

Nothing could make things harder except having to stop at the middle of the week because you ran out of idea on what to eat on the fourth or fifth day. Planning your meal and snacks for one full week gives you the buffer period to not worry about anything.

5. Get enough support

Expect the unexpected because inevitably, what you don't expect will come up. The first few weeks of your low carbohydrate diet can be hard and although it's an easy low carb diet, you still definitely need all the support you can get. The temptations are inevitable and you must accept that "speedbumps" will always be there; thus, someone should be there to help you work through these.

GETTING STARTED WITH
A LOW CARB DIET PLAN

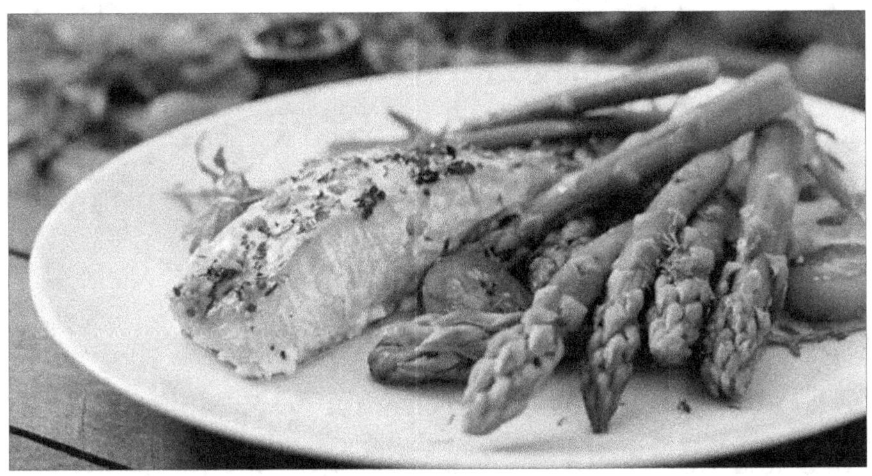

Once you've finally made the decision to lose weight, and you've decided you want to try a low carb diet plan, the hard part is practically over. All you need to do now is simply get started. So let's look at what your first several days of a low carb diet plan might be like.

Day one of your low carb diet plan should really start with some firm decisions. First you decide you will lose weight of course, and second, you decide to go with a low carb diet plan to accomplish that weight loss. Next, though, you need to choose which low carb diet plan you intend to follow. Three popular ones include the Atkins low carb diet plan, The South Beach low carb diet plan, and The Glycemic Index low carb diet plan.

Regardless of which plan you choose, the goal is to lower your daily intake of carbs, and start really losing some of the extra weight and fat your body has been holding on to. So on day one, decide which low carb diet plan you will be following and familiarize yourself with how that low carb diet plan works specifically.

Day two of your low carb diet plan will involve planning and preparation. First, you need to clear out your cabinets, pantry, fridge, and freezer. Toss out or give away any high carb, high sugar content foods that you won't be eating with your low carb diet plan.

Most low carb diet plans don't allow you to have certain foods in the first week or two on the plan, but you can gradually add those foods in later. So you may find yourself getting rid of foods you have right now that aren't overly high in carbs but aren't yet allowed for the start of your low carb diet plan. Don't despair though... many of these foods will be added back in over the next few weeks.

Next, you will want to make a list of what you will be eating for at least the next week. Include meals, snacks, and liquids, then create a shopping list for all of those items. Last but not least, you will go to the store and buy all of the foods on your list.

Taking these steps will help you get started right with the low carb diet plan of your choosing, and it will help you stick to the proper guidelines and instructions for that plan as well.

Day three of your low carb diet plan is when you will actually change the way you eat. You don't have to wait until this day to get started with your new low carb diet plan, but it can be helpful to start fresh at the beginning of a new day, instead of starting in the middle of a day. Starting your new low carb diet plan at the beginning of a brand new day will make you feel more committed to the plan instead of feeling like it was an impulsive decision on the spur of the moment.

Day three is a good day to do a bit of cooking too. By preparing foods that are allowed during this beginning stage of your low carb diet plan, you're making sure you will always have something good to eat that's easy to just grab and go. One of the biggest pitfalls of most low carb diet plans is that you need to cook the proper foods for your particular plan. And if you don't have something cooked and ready when you want it, you're more likely to fall off the plan and sabotage your weight loss efforts.

The next several days of your low carb diet plan might not be the best. You will experience sugar and starch cravings, you may be tired and lethargic, and you may have headaches or mild dizziness. These are all standard symptoms of starting a low carb diet plan because your body is cleaning out all the extra starches, sugars and junk that's been stored up for a while. Your body is going through withdrawal from the lack of sugar that it's used to, and these early days on your low carb diet plan are when having pre-cooked foods is most important because you're at a higher risk of quitting when you're not feeling well.

Once those few days of the withdrawal are over though, you will very likely be thrilled with the results of choosing a low carb diet plan. You'll have more energy, you won't feel as bloated, and you might even notice clothes are already started to fit more loosely too!

THE INS AND OUTS OF LOW CARB EATING

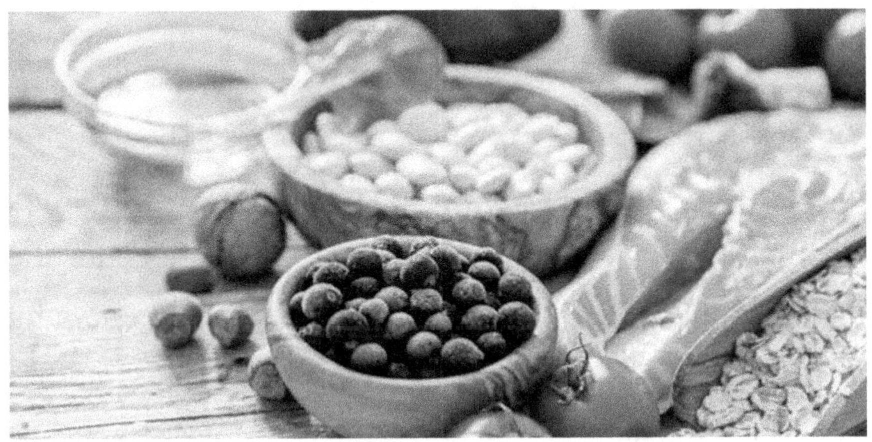

When shopping for low carb foods, it's always good to know what you are looking for so you aren't fooled by what might seem low carb but really isn't. In this article, "The Ins and Outs of low carb grocery shopping", you will understand the two different types of carbohydrates there are in foods. You are also going to see what to look for when reading food labels, and finally, I'm going to help you understand how many carbohydrates you should be eating, so let's get started!

The first thing you want to understand is the difference between the types of carbohydrate. There are two major different types of carbs in foods. They are simple and complex carbohydrate. Simple carbohydrates are also called simple sugars. Simple sugars are found in refined sugars such as candy, white table sugar, fruit, and milk. You want to get most of your simple carbs from healthier sources such as fruit and milk.

Complex carbs are also known as starches. These include grains, pasta, bread, crackers, and rice. Just as with simple carbohydrate, some choices of complex carbs are better than others. For instance, refined grains (i.e. white flour and white rice), have been processed and a lot of the nutrients and fiber have been removed.

On the flip side, unrefined grains are rich in fiber and can help your digestive system to work well. Fiber helps you to feel full, so you are less likely to eat things like junk food such as candy and chips. Of course, it's always better to get your carbs from complex carbohydrate sources than from simple. Although both types can be part of a healthy diet if you get your simple carbs from sources like fruit and milk. Candy and chips should not be part of your daily diet! Certain vegetables can also be a good source of simple carbohydrate.

When it comes to eating a low carb diet and keeping track of your carbohydrate, you want to read food labels! Knowing how to read food labels and understanding what the label is saying is very important to keeping track of how many carbs you are eating throughout the day!

This might be controversial and some people won't agree, but when you count your carbs throughout the day, you need to count total carbs, not net carbs! Here's what Web MD under Women's Health in the article "When a carb's not a carb: the net carb debate" says about counting total carbs vs. Net carbs:

In an effort to cash in on the low-carb craze, food manufacturers have invented a new category of carbohydrates known as "net carbs," which promises to let dieters eat the sweet and creamy foods they crave without suffering the carb consequences.

But the problem is that there is no legal definition of the "net," "active," or "impact" carbs popping up on food labels and advertisements. The only carbohydrate information regulated by the FDA is provided in the Nutrition Facts label, which lists total carbohydrates and breaks them down into dietary fiber and sugars.

Any information or claims about carbohydrate content that appear outside that box have not been evaluated by the FDA.

"These terms have been made up by food companies," says Wahida Karmally, DrPH, RD, director of nutrition at the Irving Center for Clinical Research at Columbia University. "It's a way for the manufacturers of these products to draw attention to them and make them look appealing by saying, 'Look, you can eat all these carbs, but you're really not impacting your health, so to speak.'"

So the bottom line is that food companies are trying to fool consumers in order to sell more of their product! That's nothing new!

So when you look at food labels and want to see how much carbohydrate is in a particular food, you want to go by the total carbohydrate. Look at the top of the label and see how many servings are in a particular food item. Then look down the label until you find carbohydrate. The amount of carbs listed on the label is per serving of that particular food item. Don't make the mistake of just looking at the food label and thinking that the whole container has x amount of carbs. It's always per serving!

When on a low carb diet, how many carbs should you be eating per day? Well, that can vary. It depends on what you're trying to accomplish. If you're trying to lose weight and are just getting started, it's probably best to eat 20 carbs or less per day for at least 2 weeks. After two weeks, you can raise the amount by small increments weekly until you are maxed out around 75 carbs per day.

If you're diabetic, there's not really one size that fits all with this. The American Diabetes Association recommends 45-60 grams of carbohydrate per meal to start with. It's also best to consume complex carbs over simple carbs. Always make sure you check with your doctor though before doing anything!

Doing your research is very important before starting a low carb diet. Again, there are many different reasons why people might eat low carb. Taking the time to find out how many carbs you should eat in your particular situation is vital for success! Don't just go into a low carb lifestyle blind! Learn what to look for on food labels, and know what kinds of foods are appropriate for your situation before going out and shopping for them.

ARE YOU RIGHT FOR THE KETO DIET?

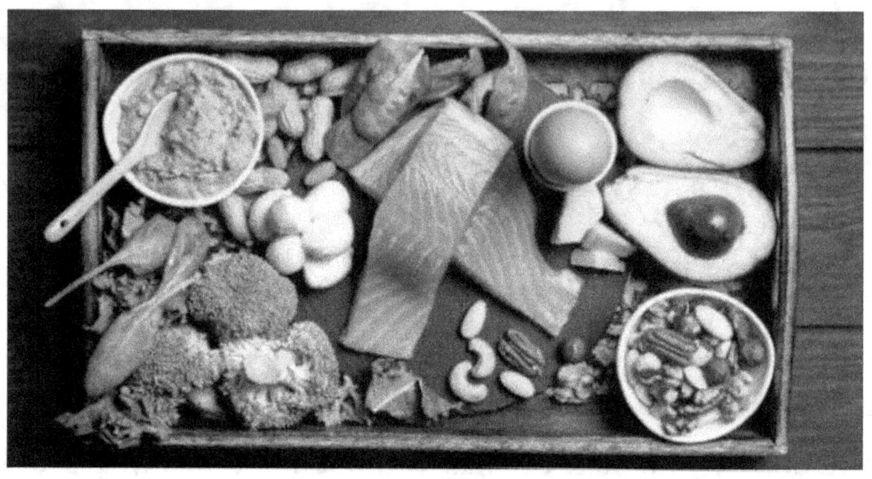

These days, it seems like everyone is talking about the ketogenic (in short, keto) diet - the very low-carbohydrate, moderate protein, a high-fat eating plan that transforms your body into a fatburning machine. Hollywood stars and professional athletes have publicly touted this diet's benefits, from losing weight, lowering blood sugar, fighting inflammation, reducing cancer risk, increasing energy, to slowing down aging. So is keto something that you should consider taking on? The following will explain what this diet is all about, the pros and cons, as well as the problems to look out for.

What Is Keto?

Normally, the body uses glucose as the main source of fuel for energy. When you are on a keto diet and you are eating very few carbs with only moderate amounts of protein (excess protein can be converted to carbs), your body switches its fuel supply to run mostly on fat. The liver produces ketones (a type of fatty acid) from fat. These ketones become a fuel source for the body, especially the brain which consumes plenty of energy and can run on either glucose or ketones.

When the body produces ketones, it enters a metabolic state called ketosis. Fasting is the easiest way to achieve ketosis. When you are fasting or eating very few carbs and only moderate amounts of protein, your body turns to burning stored fat for fuel. That is why people tend to lose more weight on the keto diet.

Benefits Of The Keto Diet

The keto diet is not new. It started being used in the 1920s as a medical therapy to treat epilepsy in children, but when anti-epileptic drugs came to the market, the diet fell into obscurity until recently. Given its success in reducing the number of seizures in epileptic patients, more and more research is being done on the ability of the diet to treat a range of neurologic disorders and other types of chronic illnesses.

Neurodegenerative diseases.

New research indicates the benefits of keto in Alzheimer's, Parkinson's, autism, and multiple sclerosis (MS). It may also be protective in traumatic brain injury and stroke. One theory for keto's neuroprotective effects is that the ketones produced during ketosis provide additional fuel to brain cells, which may help those cells resist the damage from inflammation caused by these diseases.

Obesity and weight loss

. If you are trying to lose weight, the keto diet is very effective as it helps to access and shed your body fat. Constant hunger is the biggest issue when you try to lose weight. The keto diet helps avoid this problem because reducing carb consumption and increasing fat intake promote satiety, making it easier for people to adhere to the diet. In a study, obese test subjects lost double the amount of weight within 24 weeks going on a low-carb diet (20.7 lbs) compared to the group on a low-fat diet (10.5 lbs).

Type 2 diabetes.

Apart from weight loss, the keto diet also helps enhance insulin sensitivity, which is ideal for anyone with type 2 diabetes. In a study published in Nutrition & Metabolism, researchers noted that diabetics who ate low-carb keto diets were able to significantly reduce their dependence on diabetes medication and may even reverse it eventually. Additionally, it improves other health markers such as lowering triglyceride and LDL (bad) cholesterol and raising HDL (good) cholesterol.

Cancer.

Most people are not aware that cancer cells' main fuel is glucose. That means eating the right diet may help suppress cancer growth. Since the keto diet is very low in carbs, it deprives the cancer cells of their primary source of fuel, which is sugar. When the body produces ketones, the healthy cells can use that as energy but not the cancer cells, so they are effectively being starved to death. As early as 1987, studies on keto diets have already demonstrated reduced tumor growth and improved survival for a number of cancers.

The key distinction between the keto diet and the standard American or Paleo diets is that it contains far fewer carbs and much more fat. The keto diet results in ketosis with circulating ketones ranging from 0.5-5.0 mM. This can be measured using a home blood ketone monitor with ketone test strips. (Please know that testing ketones in urine is not accurate.)

How To Formulate A Keto Diet

1. Carbohydrates

For most people, to achieve ketosis (getting ketones above 0.5 mM) requires them to restrict carbs to somewhere between 20-50 grams (g)/day. The actual amount of carbs will vary from person to person. Generally, the more insulin resistant a person is, the more resistant they are to ketosis. Some insulin sensitive athlete's exercising vigorously can consume more than 50 g/day and remain in ketosis, whereas individuals with type 2 diabetes and insulin resistance may need to be closer to 20-30 g/day.

When calculating carbs, one is allowed to use net carbs, meaning total carbs minus fiber and sugar alcohols. The concept of net carbs is to incorporate only carbs that increase blood sugar and insulin. Fiber does not have any metabolic or hormonal impact and so do most sugar alcohols. The exception is maltitol, which can have a non-trivial impact on blood sugar and insulin. Therefore, if maltitol is on the ingredient list, sugar alcohol should not be deducted from total carbs.

The level of carbs one can consume and remain in ketosis may also change over time depending on keto-adaptation, weight loss, exercise habits, medications, etc. Therefore, one should measure his/her ketone levels on a routine basis.

In terms of the overall diet, carb-dense foods like pasta, cereals, potatoes, rice, beans, sugary sweets, sodas, juices, and beer are not suitable.

Most dairy products contain carbs in the form of lactose (milk sugar). However, some have fewer carbs and can be used regularly. These include hard cheeses (Parmesan, cheddar), soft, high-fat cheeses (Brie), full-fat cream cheese, heavy whipping cream, and sour cream.

A carb level less than 50 g/day generally breaks down to the following:

- 5-10 g carbs from protein-based foods. Eggs, cheese, and shellfish will carry a few residual grams of carbs from natural sources and added marinades and spices.

- 10-15 g carbs from non-starchy vegetables.

- 5-10 g carbs from nuts/seeds. Most nuts contain 5-6 g carbs per ounce.

- 5-10 g carbs from fruits such as berries, olives, tomatoes, and avocados.

- 5-10 g carbs from miscellaneous sources such as low-carb desserts, high-fat dressings, or drinks with very small amounts of sugar.

Beverages

Most people require at least half a gallon of total fluid per day. The best sources are filtered water, organic coffee and tea (regular and decaf, unsweetened), and unsweetened almond and coconut milk. Diet sodas and drinks are best avoided as they contain artificial sweeteners. If you drink red or white wine, limit to 1-2 glasses, the dryer the better. If you drink spirits, avoid the sweetened mixed drinks.

2. Protein

A keto diet is not a high protein diet. The reason is that protein increases insulin and can be converted to glucose through a process called gluconeogenesis, hence, inhibiting ketosis.

However, a keto diet should not be too low in protein either as it can lead to loss of muscle tissue and function.

The average adult requires about 0.8-1.5 g per kilogram (kg) of lean body mass per day. It is important to make the calculation based on lean body mass, not total body weight. The reason is that fat mass does not require protein to maintain, only the lean muscle mass.

For example, if an individual weighs 150 lbs (or 150/2.2 = 68.18 kg) and has a body fat content of 20% (or lean body mass of 80% = 68.18 kg x 0.8 = 54.55 kg), the protein requirement may range from 44 (= 54.55 x 0.8) to 82 (= 54.55 x 1.5) g/day.

Those who are insulin resistant or doing the keto diet for therapeutic reasons (cancer, epilepsy, etc.) should aim to be closer to the lower protein limit. The higher limit is for those who are very active or athletic. For everyone else who is using the keto diet for weight loss or other health benefits, the amount of daily protein can be somewhere in between.

- Best sources of high quality protein include:

- Organic, pastured eggs (6-8 g of protein/egg)

- Grass-fed meats (6-9 g of protein/oz)

- Animal-based sources of omega-3 fats, such as wild-caught Alaskan salmon, sardines, and anchovies, and herrings. (6-9 g of protein/oz)

- Nuts and seeds, such as macadamia, almonds, pecans, flax, hemp, and sesame seeds. (4-8 g of protein/quarter cup)

- Vegetables (1-2 g of protein/oz)

3. Fat

Having figured out the exact amounts of carbs and protein to eat, the rest of the diet comes from fat. A keto diet is necessarily high in fat. If sufficient fat is eaten, body weight is maintained. If weigh loss is desired, one should consume less dietary fat and rely on stored body fat for energy expenditure instead.

For individuals who consume 2,000 calories a day to maintain their weight, daily fat intakes range from about 156-178 g/day. For large or very active individuals with high energy requirements who are maintaining weight, fat intakes may even exceed 300 g/day.

Most people can tolerate high intakes of fat, but certain conditions such as gallbladder removal may affect the amount of fat that can be consumed at a single meal. In which case, more frequent meals or use of bile salts or pancreatic enzymes high in lipase may be helpful.

Avoid eating undesirable fats such as trans fat, highly refined polyunsaturated vegetable oils, as well as high amounts of omega-6 polyunsaturated fats.

Best foods to obtain high-quality fats include:

- Avocados and avocado oil

- Coconuts and coconut oil

- Grass-fed butter, ghee, and beef fat

- Organic, pastured heavy cream

- Olive oil

- Lard from pastured pigs

- Medium chain triglycerides (MCTs) MCT is a specific type of fat that is metabolized differently from regular long-chain fatty acids. The liver can use MCTs to rapidly produce energy, even before glucose, thus allowing increased production of ketones.

Concentrated sources of MCT oil are available as supplements. Many people use them to help achieve ketosis. The only food that is uniquely high in MCTs is coconut oil. About two-thirds of the coconut fat is derived from MCT.

Who Should Be Cautious With A Keto Diet?

For most people, a keto diet is very safe. However, there are certain individuals who need to take special care and discuss with their doctors before going on such a diet.

- Those taking medications for diabetes. Dosage may need to be adjusted as blood sugar goes down with a low-carb diet.

- Those taking medications for high blood pressure. Dosage may need to be adjusted as blood pressure goes down with a low-carb diet.

- Those who are breastfeeding should not go on a very strict low-carb diet as the body can lose about 30 g of carbs per day via the milk. Therefore, have at least 50 g of carbs per day while breastfeeding.

- Those with kidney disease should consult with their doctors before doing a keto diet.

- Common Concerns With A Keto Diet

- Not being able to reach ketosis. Make sure you are not eating too much protein and there are no hidden carbs in the packaged foods that you consume.

- Eating the wrong kinds of fat such as the highly refined polyunsaturated corn and soybean oils.

Symptoms of a "keto-flu", such as feeling light-headed, dizziness, headaches, fatigue, brain fog, and constipation. When in ketosis, the body tends to excrete more sodium. If one is not getting enough sodium from the diet, symptoms of a keto-flu may appear. This is easily remedied by drinking 2 cups of broth (with added salt) per day. If you exercise vigorously or the sweat rate is high, you may need to add back even more sodium.

Dawn effect. Normal fasting blood sugars are less than 100 mg/dl and most people in ketosis will achieve this level if they are not diabetic. However, in some people fasting blood sugars tend to increase, especially in the morning, while on a keto diet. This is called the "dawn effect" and is due to the normal circadian rise in morning cortisol (stress hormone) that stimulates the liver to make more glucose. If this happens, make sure you are not consuming excessive protein at dinner and not too close to bedtime. Stress and poor sleep can also lead to higher cortisol levels. If you are insulin resistant, you may also need more time to achieve ketosis.

Low athletic performance. Keto-adaptation usually takes about 4 weeks. During which, instead of doing intense workouts or training, switch to something that is less vigorous. After the adaptation period, athletic performance usually returns to normal or even better, especially for endurance sports.

Keto-rash is not a common side effect of the diet. Probable causes include the production of acetone (a form of ketone) in the sweat that irritates the skin or nutrient deficiencies including protein or minerals. Shower immediately after exercise and make sure you eat nutrient dense whole foods.

Ketoacidosis. This is a very rare condition that occurs when blood ketone levels go above 15 mM. A well-formulated keto diet does not cause ketoacidosis. Certain conditions such as type 1 diabetes, being on medications with SGLT-2 inhibitors for type 2 diabetes, or breastfeeding require extra caution. Symptoms include lethargy, nausea, vomiting, and rapid shallow breathing. Mild cases can be resolved using sodium bicarbonate mixed with diluted orange or apple juice. Severe symptoms require prompt medical attention.

Is Keto Safe For Long-Term?

This is an area of some controversy. Though there have not been any studies indicating any adverse long-term effects of being on a keto diet, many experts now believe that the body may develop a "resistance" to the benefits of ketosis unless one regularly cycles in and out of it. In addition, eating a very high-fat diet in the long-term may not be suitable for all body types.

Cyclical keto diet

Once you are able to generate over 0.5 mM of ketones in the blood on a consistent basis, it is time to start reintroducing carbs back into the diet. Instead of eating merely 20-50 g of carbs/day, you may want to increase it to 100-150 g on those carb-feeding days. Typically, 2-3 times a week will be sufficient. Ideally, this is also done on strength training days on which you actually increase your protein intake.

This approach of cycling may make the diet plan more acceptable to some people who are reluctant to permanently eliminate some of their favorite foods. However, it may also lower resolve and commitment to the keto diet or trigger binges in susceptible individuals.

3 TIPS FOR AN ENJOYABLE LOW CARB DIET

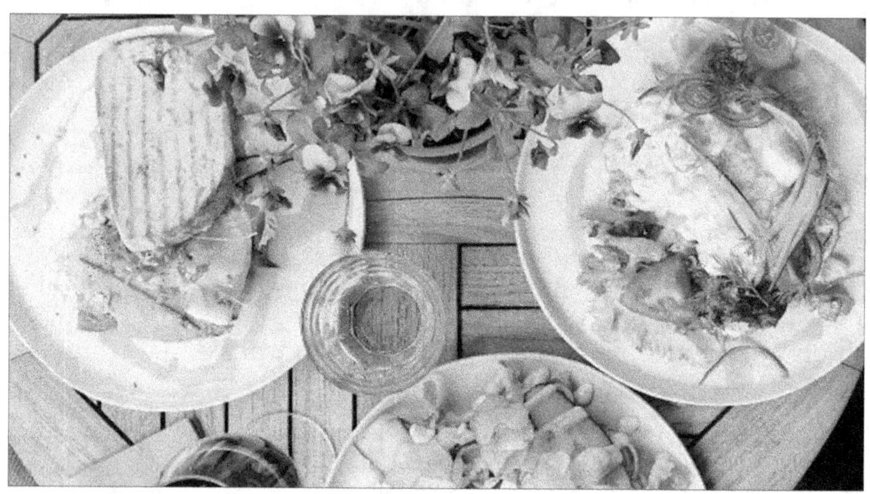

There is a wide variety of food choices that a low carb dieter can enjoy. All you need is to grab a good low carb cookbook and prepare a menu that you will enjoy. Here are some tips that you can keep in mind for a more enjoyable low carb diet.

1. Enjoying Your Breakfast

You can enjoy your regular bacon and eggs breakfast even if you are on the low carb diet. Just make sure that your bacon is not cured. You can also choose from the other regular breakfast foods that a low carb dieter can pursue. This includes ricotta cheese that you can make into a porridge with soya bran. You can also have cereal or granola if you need a quick breakfast.

2. *Sumptuous Meals*

You can also enjoy a good amount of meat in your low carb food diet. Your life need not revolve on vegetables, fruits, flax bread or salad. You can still enjoy the meat you love. Just be sure to grill or barbecue your meat, poultry or fish. This is to stay away from the harmful fats of cooking with oil. Also, be sure to choose the ones that are not cured to stay away from carcinogenic elements.

3. *Bring Along a Healthy Snack*

Most dieters think that they can only stick to the salad if they have to eat low carb foods. However, a good serving of a sandwich will not be bad every now and then. All you need is to prepare properly the menu for the serving. Instead of the regular pieces of bread that you used to eat, you can make use of the low carb bread in your menu. Bread made from flax and whole wheat is good for your recipes.

Sticking to your low carb food diet may be one of the best decisions that you can stand firm with. You need not worry with this, as you have the choice to make your mealtime as enjoyable as you want it to be.

The truth is that no matter how motivated and willing to lose weight we may be, it is still a difficult task to accomplish. If you've chosen a Low-Carb diet plan, these nine Low Carb diet tips will help you in achieving your goals easier.

- Carbohydrates should only amount to 10% of your daily calorie intake. Eat plenty of fruits and vegetables according to what's allowed in your chosen Low Carb diet. Also, include protein in your diet.

- Every Low-Carb diet has its own set of rules. Do not mix Low Carb diet plans. Follow the guidelines as outlined to ensure your success.

- Avoid foods with white flour and/or sugar. Eat whole grain bread that allows for easier digestion, and give you a full feeling faster. Sweets will only make you crave more sweets.

- Beware of hidden sugars in carbohydrates. Certain carbs convert to sugar faster, like certain fruits and veggies such as carrots. Try to stick to low sugar carbs.

- Take fiber supplements, as well as vitamin and mineral supplements. The fiber will aid in digestion while making you feel full. The vitamins and minerals will supplement for a balanced, healthy diet.

- Caffeine is a strong stimulant that increases the hunger pangs in some people. Cut down on caffeine, and preferably drink decaffeinated coffee.

- Drink plenty of water. Drinking one full 8oz glass of water before every meal, will make you feel fuller and eat fewer foods. Besides this benefit, drinking at least 8 quarts of water a day will help your overall in keeping a healthy body.

- Keep on learning everything you can about the carb content in foods as well as how to mix and match foods correctly for faster weight loss and tastier meals. There are plenty of books with great low carb recipes to give you plenty of ideas.

- Visit your physician before starting a diet, and during the process of losing weight. A good plan should be supervised by a medical practitioner.

Not all Low Carb diets were created equal. Successful weight loss depends on many factors, and one of the primary ones is choosing the right Low Carb diet for you according to your lifestyle, budget and food preferences, among several other choices. Once you have chosen the right Low

Carb diet for you, these Low Carb diet tips will help you achieve success.

TIPS FOR COOKING
LOW CARB

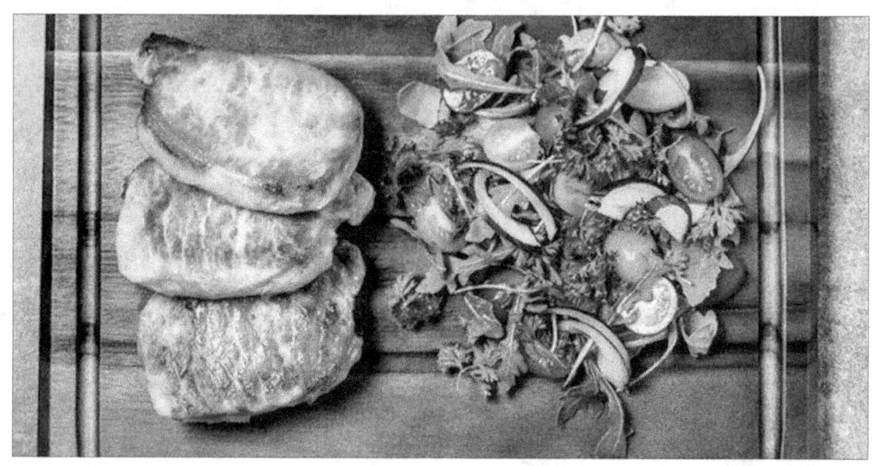

If you are committed to the low carb way of eating, but also craving some of your old comfort foods you may still be able to satisfy those cravings with a little bit of creative substitution. Some of the foods that you used to know and love have a low carb alternative available - the taste might be a little bit different but you will soon get used to that and be well on your way to happier and healthier eating!

<u>**Here are some tips you can use to make your low carb cooking easier and tastier:**</u>

- Make low carb bread crumbs for breaded foods. Foods like chicken Parmesan and stuffed peppers need to have bread crumbs to have that full taste. While you may be able to buy low carb bread crumbs, you can also make them by using low carb bread. Simply toast the low carb bread in the oven on a cookie sheet. Once it is hard, grind it up in the food processor or blender.

- Use soy flour or bake mix. When you need to use flour for baking or coating breaded foods, substitute soy flour or a baking mix like Atkins bake mix. You can convert your favorite recipes that use white flour to use these.

- Use low carb chocolate bars for cookies and muffins. Now that you've converted your favorite chocolate chip cookie recipe using soy flour, you don't want to put in those high carb chocolate chips. Chop up a low carb chocolate bar into small pieces and use that instead.

- Use Splenda instead of sugar. Recipes that call for sugar can be modified to use Splenda instead. It is much lighter so you will have to experiment with it and it may not work for everything but it does bake up nice for the most part.

- Make great smoothies with low carb yogurt. Ok, well it's not technically cooking, but if you love smoothies you can make them with low carb yogurt and fruit. Just make sure you use fruit that is low in carbs and the whole fruit, not the juice as the fiber will help keep down the net carbs. Check my site below for a list of low carb fruits. Add a dash of vanilla or flavored syrup to the smoothie for added flavor.

- For a great low carb pasta substitute use spaghetti squash. We all know that low carb pasta tastes horrible so why not try a food that is low in carbs and natural too. Cut the squash in half and bake at 400 degrees F for about 40 minutes. The squash will scrape out in strings and gives the texture and feel of spaghetti. Trust me, it tastes a lot better than the low carb pasta and has about 7 grams carbs per 1 cup serving.

YOUR GUIDE TO QUICK TO FIX, EASY LOW CARB RECIPES

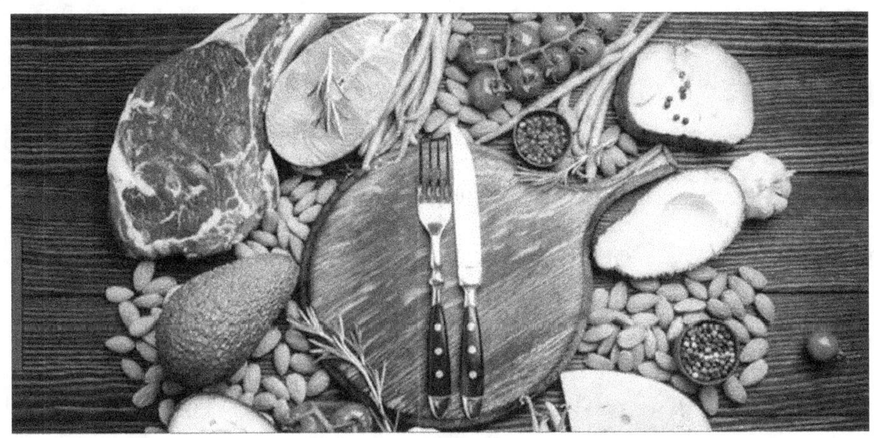

Everyone these days wants to find easy, low-carb recipes to build a healthy diet that is low in carbohydrates. With the recent low-carb craze, dieters can find information all over the place. Here are some guidelines to help you get what you want out of the low-carb phenomenon.

Whether you are searching the Internet, paging through a cookbook or digging through a friend's pile of recipes, you need to keep in mind what it is that you want out of this diet. You should desire low-carb recipes that appeal to you, that will help you lose weight healthily, that you want to eat and that you can prepare without too big a headache.

Just because foods are low-carb and diet-friendly doesn't mean they have to be bad or boring. You can find easy, low-carb recipes without sacrificing the foods you enjoy. You can easily find recipes focusing on meat, poultry or seafood. You can find dozens of great ideas for bread, pasta, sauces, and dips, as well as low-carb desserts and snacks. You can even have a low-carb beer and other alcoholic beverages.

When preparing meals containing meats, be sure to choose carefully. As you make an effort to avoid carbohydrates, you will naturally move toward foods higher in protein. Many of these high-protein foods are our favorite meats, but many of these meats are also contain large amounts of fat. To get the best out of your diet, choose easy, low-carb recipes that call for lean meat, poultry or seafood. Even lean cuts of pork are better for you than meats like bacon and beef.

Bread is another area of interest in a low-carb diet. People are often surprised to learn that cutting loaves of bread out of their diet entirely is unnecessary. With an assault on carbohydrates in their diets, many people see bread as off limits. Books have even been written discussing how to live without bread.

Bread themselves are not bad, but some can certainly not low in carbohydrates. Many easy, lowcarb recipes are available that allow you to enjoy sandwiches, burgers, toast or muffins. These recipes use a slightly different list of ingredients, but they yield healthy, tasty bread. Also, bread contains fiber, which is important to include in your diet.

Many recipes targeting a low-carb audience will specify nutritional information for the food, especially carbohydrate, protein and fiber content. This information is provided for a reason: as you probably know, foods low in carbohydrates and high in protein are central to the Atkins and other low-carb diets. Fiber is also a big part of the equation; simply put, you can have more carbs in your diet if they are in the form of fiber. Also, foods high in fiber are generally full of "good carbs," the type of carbohydrates you don't need to eliminate from your diet.

This brings up another good point: you don't need to completely eliminate carbohydrates from your diet. Keeping some carbs in your diet is healthy and does not negatively affect your diet. Most low-carb recipes have at least some carbs. Instead of cutting out all carbohydrates, you should focus on minimizing or eliminating "empty carbs," carbohydrates that come from foods with little or no nutritional value. Soft drinks and candy bard have empty carbs; fruits and vegetables, for example, have good carbs.

An important part of a low-carb diet is variety. You're trying to limit carbohydrates, but that doesn't mean you should eat eggs every day and avoid bread like the plague. Abide by the guidelines for a healthy, low-carb diet: limit but don't eliminate carbs, get plenty of fiber, make sure your protein-rich meats are not too full of fat.

Again, to easily sustain a healthy, low-carb lifestyle you should eat foods you enjoy. Low-carb foods should not be a burden. The list of diet-friendly choices has enough variety to make even the pickiest eaters happy. You have plenty of delicious, easy, low-carb recipes to choose from

LOW CARB FOODS LIST FOR A NATURALLY LOW CARB DIET

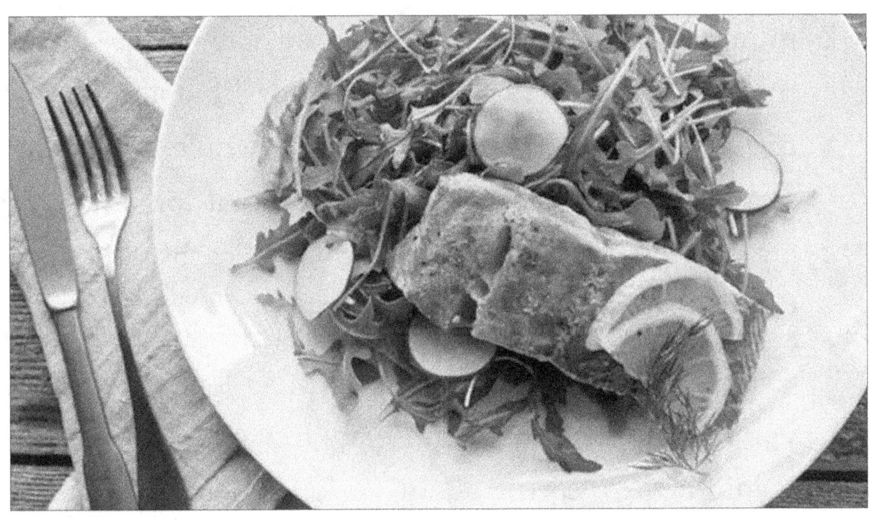

When shopping for low carb foods it seems that many of the products available are not natural, but fake versions of foods we are used to eating. How about a list of all natural, low carb foods from Mother Nature? Everyone needs to eat carbohydrates, even those on a low carb diet, so make them good carbs, complex carbohydrates from the natural, whole foods in this list.

1. Lettuce, spinach and other leafy greens are superbly natural, low carb foods. One serving (about a cup and a

half) delivers only 3 grams of carbohydrates, and those are good carbs. Cabbage, red or green, add about 5 grams to a low carb diet.

2 . Tomatoes are surprisingly low in carbohydrates. For example, 1 medium size vine ripe tomato includes 7 grams of carbohydrates. Now, that may alarm some of the fanatical low carb diet tabulators, but think about this, how many times do you eat a whole tomato in a serving? Most of the time when you eat tomatoes, you are only getting about 3 or 4 grams of carbs, and again, those are complex carbohydrates.

3 . Carrots pack so much nutrition in so few calories that you have to include them in any low carb food salad. 1 medium, raw carrot about 7" long yields 8 grams of carbohydrates. If you are only eating part of the carrot, subtract accordingly.

4 . Broccoli is a member of the cruciferous family and offers superb nutrition for a low carb diet. 1 whole medium stalk of broccoli serves up only 8 grams of very high quality, complex carbs from a whole food source. This is one fantastic, all natural, low carb food that Mother Nature intends for you to eat all the time.

5 . Green beans are some of the lowest of the low carb foods in the bean category. While black beans, red bean, Garbanzo beans, and lima beans pack almost 30 grams of

carbohydrates into a serving, green beans float in at only 5 grams of carbs per 3/4 cup serving. So, keep the beans green for a lean, mean, low carb diet machine.

6. Green peas, snow peas, and sugar snap peas are relatively low in carbs for natural foods with as much flavor. You may enjoy a half-cup of green peas, a full cup of snow peas or a cup of steamed sugar snap peas and stay fit with only about 10 grams of carbohydrates per serving, plus good fiber, which is also important for a low carbohydrate diet.

7. Cucumbers are ideal, naturally low carb foods because they are easy to clean, cut, and eat. One-third of a medium size cucumber only includes only about 3 grams of carbs.

8. Bean Sprouts are perfect for salads and in Chinese food. Even your low carb diet will certainly allow you to gobble up a full cup of bean sprouts with only 6 grams of carbs.

9. Celery is something you can never eat too much because of the fiber, the nutrients and the benefits it offers for cleansing bad breath. Also, celery is a natural, low carb food with only 3 grams of carbohydrates in 2 medium stalks.

1 0 . This last suggestion may sound a bit strange, but if you change the way you think about nutrition and the way you approach a low carb diet, then you will experience amazing results. Modern technology has made it possible for us to consume natural, low carb diet foods that are concentrated with nutrients from Mother Nature and pre-packaged for easy, convenient use. These innovative formulas are perfect for a low carb diet and made entirely from food grade herbs, not medicinal herbs, so they are very safe. You will not find these all-natural low carb foods at the grocery store or your local health food store, but they are available from cyberspace right to your door, thanks to the Internet.

No matter where you get your foods and health drinks for a low carb diet, if you stay close to nature and out of the low carb, junk food aisle you will be that much closer to perfect health and fitness.

PLANNING YOUR LOW CARB MENUS

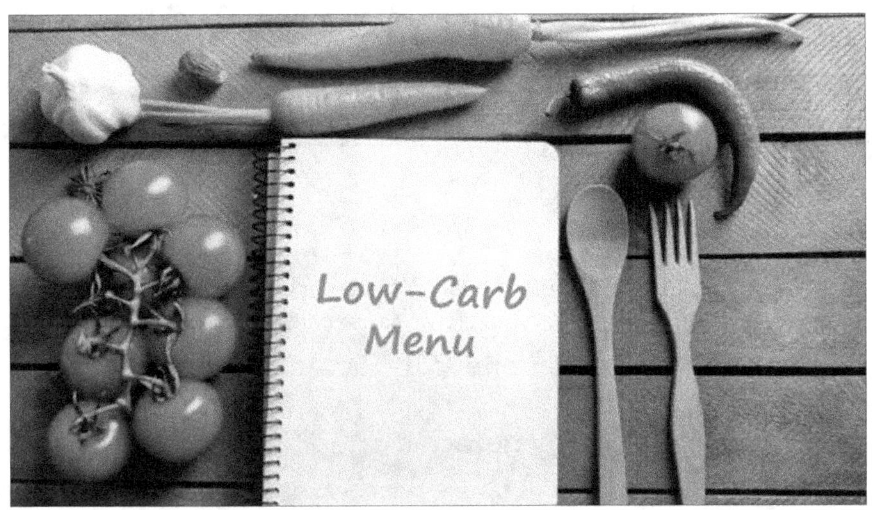

When you are new to a low carbohydrate diet it is very important to make your own low carb menus. Creating your own menus will help you reach your weight loss goal or any goal you choose when starting your new diet.

Most people never reach their weight loss goal. To have a goal and plan is the key to success when you want to lose weight. If you put your goal and plan to pen with a paper, your chance of success highly increases. Writing down your goals and plans also help you stay focused. Planning your meals is a very important part of your weight loss plan.

Before starting to plan your meals, write down your goals on paper. If you had a magic lamp with a jinn inside that could fulfill any desire, how much would you weigh? Let that be your main goal, rather than choosing something less desirable because it is easier to achieve. Also write down ten partial goals such as:

- Goal 1: Weight less than 200 pounds

- Goal 2: Loosing 5 pounds by December 1st

- Goal 3: Fit into my new coat

Now that you have written down your goals, you are ready to start planning your low carb menus. You can collect recipes that you like in your own database, document or on this cookbook. When you have collected enough recipes you start composing your menus.

It does not have to be complicated. You can generally eat an omelet for breakfast every day, chicken salad with avocado or leftovers for lunch and homemade low carbohydrate bread for my evening meal. For dinner, you can use a variety of recipes you have found online or in my cookbook. Good luck with planning your low carb menus!

We are now going to look at a typical low Carb diet meal plan for the day. It is important to note that by eating smaller portions, more regularly, is much more effective at losing weight and burning fat compared to only eating 3 meals in the day. It is also important to note that it also depends on how active you are in your day.

A Typical Daily Low Carb Menu Diet Plan
Breakfast

Breakfast is the most important meal of the day. After an 8 hour gap with no food or water, it is important to 'Break the Fast'. A good start would be a small portion of porridge with some kind of berry, like Blueberries, Strawberries or Blackberries.

An alternative could be Scrambled Eggs on Seeded or Granary Bread. A good complement would be to make up a smoothie with 3-5 different fruits. The fruit is a great choice for breakfast as it has natural sugars and it is also quick to digest, starting your day off awake and full of energy.

Low Carb Diet Snacks

Mid-morning snacks could include a Piece of Fruit, Some Mixed Nuts, Vegetables like Carrots dipped in Humus.

Lunch

Like breakfast, lunch is a very important meal. Aim to have a small fist-sized portion of Carbohydrates like Jacket Potato, Brown Rice, Wholemeal Bread, etc. A portion of protein like Chicken Breast, Cottage Cheese, Eggs, etc and a mixed portion of Vegetables.

For some people eating vegetables may be completely new. If you were brought up not eating vegetables then chances are you will be the same. A good plan is to have your salad or vegetables as a starter. Just before you start to cook, make yourself a salad including some mixed leaves, avocado, peppers, cucumber, tomatoes and splash a bit of balsamic vinegar over the top.

Dinner

If you are wanting to keep your low Carb diet foods to a minimum then simply just replace your complex Carbs with more fruit and vegetables. Again if you try to have a portion of each food group, you will be on a great track. There is no one low Carb menu diet plan that should be set in stone. I think it is important to make a low Carb diet a way of life and the sooner you can make it a habit, the easier it will be.

LOW CARB SNACKS THAT KIDS AND ADULTS WILL LOVE

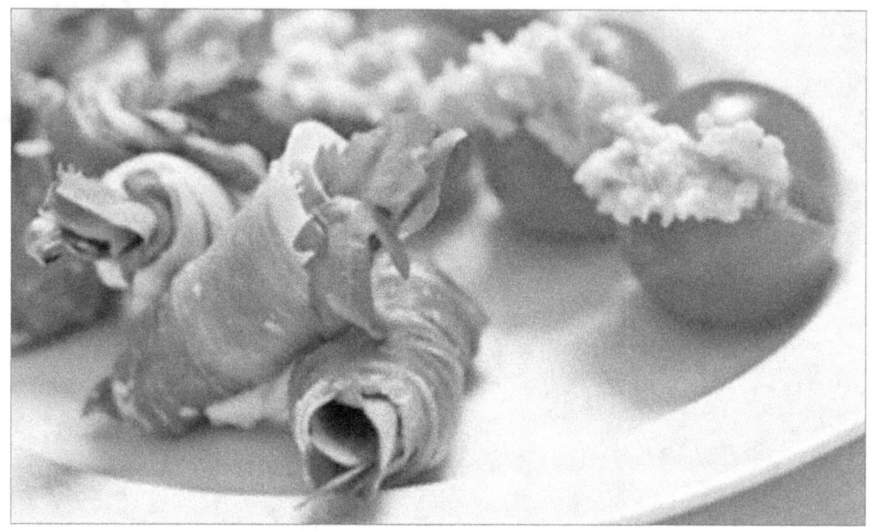

It's the highlight of any school day - recess. This is applicable to any grade-schooler. But as parents, we pretty much have to put healthy and low-carb snacks in our children's lunch boxes. Bear in mind that when a kid gains weight at such a young age, he will have a difficult time shedding the excess pounds when he gets older.

Cakes, candied cereals, ice cream, flavored popcorn, cookies, candies, muffins and all kinds of pastries may seem so appealing. I bet your mouth is watering simply by reading that passage. Sure these are low in fat but take note, these are relatively high in calories.

But there is a way for us to satisfy our sweet tooth craving the Low Carb Way. First of all, you must have the control to not reach in for the chips and crackers in between meals, or else you're engaging in a low-carb diet will turn out to be completely pointless.

A low carb snack must ideally have healthy fat, protein, and fiber. If you are having eggs or jerky, you might as well have vegetables with it.

Here's a rundown of low-carb snacks you can consider munching on:

- Celery with tuna salad

- Celery with peanut butter

- Hard-boiled eggs

- Pickles and cheddar cheese

- Berries and cottage cheese

- Nuts. Best serve when kept in the freezer.

- Sunflower seeds

- Pumpkin seeds

- Jerky-like turkey or beef. Find the low-sugar variety

- Shakes. Make sure it's low carb though

- Cheese sticks

- Sugar-free Jello

- Apple slices

- Sugar-free yogurt flavored with berries

- Lettuce roll-ups on luncheon meat, tuna, or egg salad

- Lettuce dipped in bean dip, spinach dip or another low carb dip

- Ricotta cheese with nuts, fruit or seeds

- Mushroom and cheese spread

- Low carb snack bars

Take note though that just because these are low-carbohydrate, these snacks are healthy. It may be popular and has already dominated the snack food companies and market but as a consumer, you must still be careful when choosing the low-carb snacks you will provide yourself and your family.

First off, low carb snack bars. There are tons of snack bars to choose from in the grocery. Not all of them provide good nutrition. Some low carb snack bars are there to maintain phases of low carb diets because they still contain calories. The sugar they have to contain alcohol. Alcohol sugars in low carb snack bars will be difficult to digest and result in gas.

If you choose to settle for low-carb cookie mixes, then the best we can recommend is the lowcarb chocolate chip cookies mix and the low-carb peanut butter cookies mix. Simply because peanut butter is already an example of a low-carb snack and chocolate chip cookies' sugar content is balanced out with the help of the eggs and butter (light) mix.

If you would like to try out low carb shakes, make sure to read the labels so you will have an idea of the nutritional content. Double check if the shake mix is low on glycemic.

As pointed out by Dr. Robert Atkins in his Atkins diet, the cause of weight gain is "stodgy" food like bread and potatoes. More often than not, dieters trying out the low-carb diet often complain that they miss eating bread. If it is any consolation, there are some low carb bread out there in the market. These low carb bread have added soy flour to the mix.

But that does not mean that this bread is wheat free. They are also not gluten-free. So the best way for you to achieve success in the low-carb diet is to not eat bread entirely. Yeah, you will miss it but it is for the best.

Now, if you feel that you have been very good at sticking with your low-carb diet and deserve to have a binge day once in a while, you can do so. Does pizza sound good? Well, glad to inform you that there is low-carb crust pizza with healthy toppings that is most suitable for the low-carb dieter. Fresh marinara on pizza sauce added with goat cheese, basil, vegetables, and tomatoes are enough for a dieter's mouth to water.

Being on a low-carb diet does not mean that you will repress yourself, it only means you have to regulate what you put in your mouth.

WHAT ARE THE BENEFITS OF THE LOW-CARB DIET?

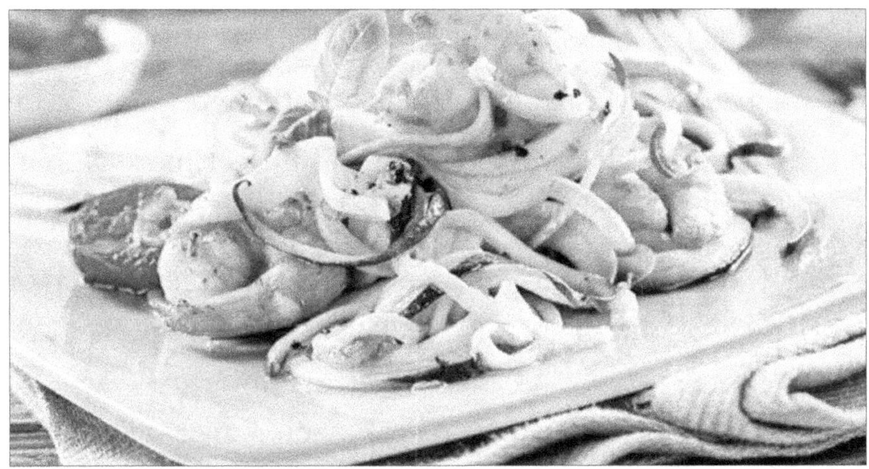

Are you one of those who hate dieting? Well, you are not alone, almost all of us hate the deprivation from food that dieting brings to us. Aside from the fact that our parents raise us to believe that food intake is necessary to keep us energetic, especially carbohydrates. Potatoes and bread are the essential members of our diet from morning, noon and night. Therefore, we resent the idea that carbohydrates are not good for us.

However, your thinking might change upon reading the low-carb diet overview. In the low-carb diet overview, you will learn that energy does not come from carbohydrates alone.

Low-carb diet overview will also tell you that good fats convert to energy much like carbohydrates, as we know it to be. Low-carb diet overview will likewise tell you about the recommended carbohydrates like whole grain, fruits, and vegetables. However, you should minimize the intake of carbohydrates to as low as 10% of your total calorie intake. If you can maintain your consumption of carbohydrates to as low as 10% of your calorie intake, you should eat more fats and moderate protein. Then, the low-carb diet overview will be the best tool to complement your weight loss regimen and avoid jumping on the obese bandwagon.

The low-carb diet overview will explain how you can best manage your weight. In contrast with the belief that carbohydrates are necessary to build your energy profile, fat may replace carbohydrates in this arena.

You will also learn from the low-carb diet overview that it is the best diet for obese individuals. Diabetics may also use the low-carb diet overview to combat the cause of obesity, high cholesterol, high blood pressure, hypoglycemia, and type II diabetes because studies show that low-carb diet attacks the condition called hyperinsulinemia. Hyperinsulinemia is a condition where insulin levels in the blood are elevated.

It may also be helpful knowledge you will get from a low-carb diet overview is the advantages one will get from a low-carb diet. Sustained weight loss is one advantage of a low-carb diet. Another advantage you will learn from low-carb diet overview and low-carb dieting is stable blood sugar; this is specifically important for diabetics and those people prone to diabetes. If you have a relative who is a diabetic, then you are one of those people prone to diabetes. Low cholesterol level is also an advantage of low-carb dieting. Some low-carb dieters also report being more energetic than their counterparts who are not dieting.

Finally, here are some basic guidelines you will get from the low-carb diet overview. You should limit your carbohydrates intake to 10% or less of your total calorie intake. You will also find the list of allowed foods, you will also find the list of foods to avoid and foods with hidden sugar in the low-carb diet overview. Avoiding food containing sugar and white flour is also part of the low carb diet. Avoiding caffeine and drinking lots of clean and clear water also helps in the dieting process. Taking fiber supplements and vitamin will help during the initial stage of lowcarb dieting.

LOW CARBS DIETS
HOW TO MAKE THEM WORK

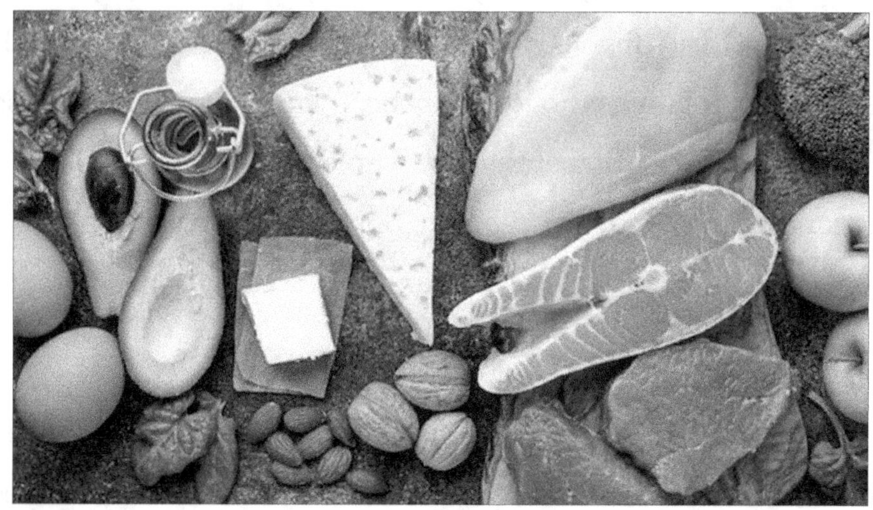

If you have lived on this planet, you have probably heard about Low Carbs Diets. But what exactly are low carbs diets? Are they healthy or not? There are different opinions among the nutrition and weight loss expert if this kind of diet is healthy and what effect does it have on your body.

The basic principle of all Low Carbs Diets is to reduce the number of carbohydrates you take in on a daily basis. What happens with carbohydrates in our bodies? Glucose causes blood sugar to rise and increases the production of insulin. The function of the insulin is to hook up with glucose and takes it to the cells which are used for energy. The amount of glucose which is not used is stored as glycogen for future energy requirements or it is stored as fat.

If you look at these facts, it's simple math. If you use more energy than you take it in with carbohydrates, you will lose weight. But it is not as simple as it may look. Reducing the carbs in your daily routine is just one step to lose weight and to become healthier. The other necessary step is to take exercise. Exercise is a vital step in the process. With exercise, you will take your body into a higher gear and the requirement for energy in your body will increase, so the body is forced to take the additional energy from a different source - fat. That means, with the right approach that we are on the right track and we can start with our Low Carbs Diets.

With reducing the intake of the carbohydrates and taking the regular exercise we are on a good way to lose weight. The more consistent we are and the more exercise we will do, the more weight we will lose. And the best thing is that we will be happy with ourselves and happy with the fact that we did something useful for our body. On the internet, you will find a lot of different Low Carbs Diets and you have to find the one that is most suitable for your lifestyle and the one that you will really enjoy. If you do that you have made your first and the most important step in achieving your goals. Be happy with yourself and the low carbs diets you choose and you will succeed.

LOSE WEIGHT
THE LOW CARB WAY

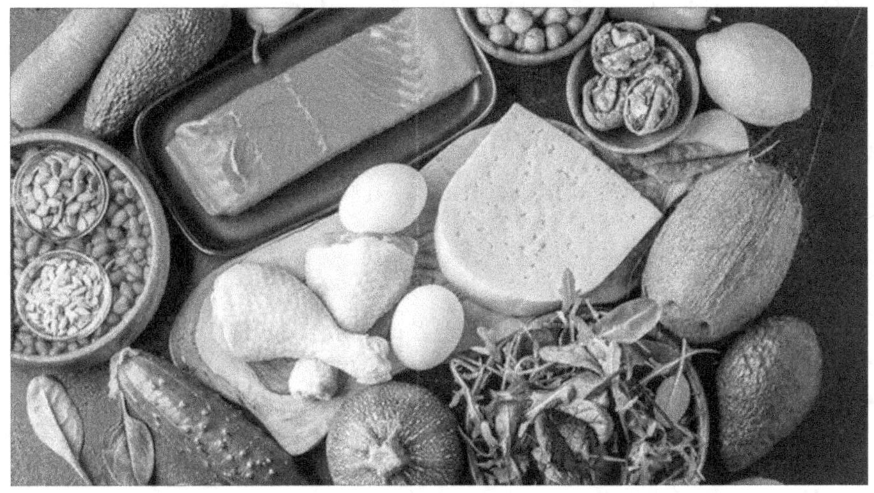

If you want to lose weight or need to become healthier, you might want to consider eating low carb. Losing weight the low carb way is a healthy way to not only slim down, but eating low carb can help with other ailments you might have.

You may have tried every diet in the book from Weight Watchers to Jenny Craig to using Slim Fast along with many others, and none of them worked for you. And it's really no wonder. What these fad diets and products include, are high carbs! All you have to do is check out the labels on them and you'll see!

Not to mention, the USDA daily food guide pyramid states that at least 60% of our daily caloric intake should come from carbohydrate! The fact of the matter is that sugar and carbohydrate help put on and store the pounds! So why in the world would a weight loss product be full of carbohydrate? It's so these companies can continue to sell you their product - simple.

Yes, our bodies need some carbohydrate, but in order to lose weight, you need to lower your carb intake along with your calories.

Don't fall for the false belief that if you lower your carbs, you can pig out and eat over the top! A lot of people try that and end up wondering why they start gaining weight!

Losing weight the low carb way means lowering your carbohydrate intake by choosing foods low in carbohydrate and eating normal sized or smaller portions. It's a good idea to keep track of not only the number of carbs you are taking in per day but the number of calories also.

Depending on how much weight you are trying to lose, depends on how many carbs you want to start out restricting from your diet.

Other key elements to low carb weight loss are staying hydrated and making sure you are getting enough protein. You are definitely going to want to increase your protein intake when you lower your carb intake. You also want to increase your water intake. Doing so will help you to not become dehydrated.

The reason lowering your carbohydrate intake helps you to lose weight is found in the reasoning of when people become overweight, it's because of something called hyperinsulinemia. This is elevated insulin levels in the blood.

When you eat a high carb meal, the higher blood sugar increases insulin production by the pancreas. (Insulin is the hormone that allows blood sugar into our cells). Insulin also allows fat to be deposited and signals hunger to the brain! So you end up eating more and more carbohydrate which in turn causes more insulin to be released which in turn causes more fat to be stored.

As time goes by, your cells become resistant to insulin and your pancreas has to work harder, producing 4 to 5 times the amount of insulin just to keep with the demand being placed on it. Obviously, that's not good and can cause many different health issues.

Putting a halt to this entire carbohydrate intake stops the vicious cycle. When you lower your carb intake, your insulin levels will decrease and your glucagon levels will increase. Glucagon is another hormone in the body that causes body fat to be burned.

So changing your eating habits by eating a low carb diet can help you lose weight and become healthier. There's really no drawback at all from losing weight the low carb way!

If you've been eating high carb and are overweight, please take the time to delve further into this way of eating. It can only improve your health and add years to your life.

LOSE WEIGHT THROUGH LOW CARB DIETING

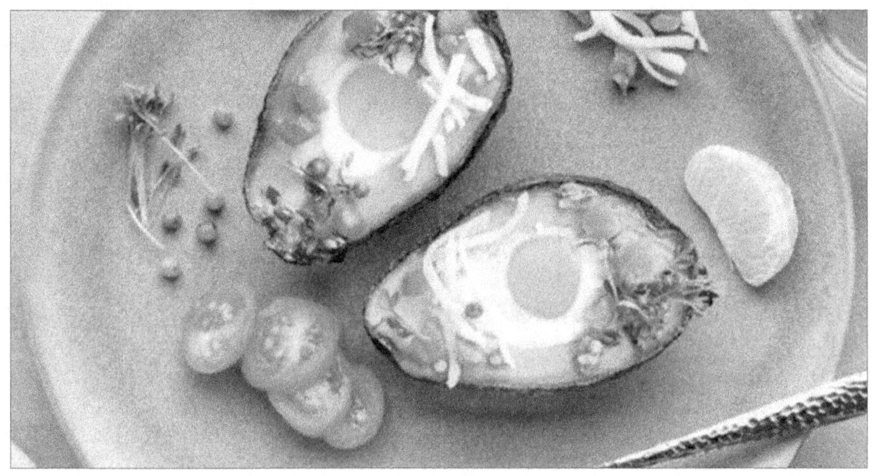

Low carbohydrate diets have recently become quite popular, particularly after the publication of the Atkins diet. Many people want to lose some weight, and it seems like all of them want a quick and easy way to do it. Some people might need to lose 100 pounds for medical reasons, while others get stressed about a few pounds, even though they don't really need to lose any weight.

There are many different diets to choose from, including low carbohydrate diets. The fact is, most diets will lead to weight loss if they're followed properly. This does not mean you need to do everything the diet says every moment of every single day. How you deal with the inevitable slip up - times when you eat excessively or feast on foods that aren't on your diet - is far more important. If you're able to overlook these mistakes and get back onto your diet plan without giving yourself a hard time, you'll probably succeed in losing weight. Everyone has days like that, but it's essential to let them go and accept them as just another step on your path to permanent weight loss.

You also need to find a diet that's easy to follow. The rules of low carb diets are simple, so they suit many people. Just like the name implies, a low carb diet consists of eliminating or restricting your consumption of high carbohydrate foods, including pasta, bread, potatoes, rice, and other grains, as well as foods that contain sugar. It's easy to eat meals that avoid these high carb foods once you understand what they are.

Low carb diets do receive some criticism, mainly based on the fact that dieters receive most of their daily calories from dairy, meat and other high foods high in fat. Consuming high amounts of saturated fats can lead to high cholesterol and related health issues. For this reason, a dieter should seek the advice of his or her physician before beginning a low carb diet. Weight loss sometimes progresses well in the early stages of a diet, but some people cannot handle the longterm dietary restrictions and begin to deviate from their diet.

Eliminating bread and pasta is one of the most difficult obstacles for many people following a low carb diet. Many foods that are quick to prepare should be eliminated because they're based on carbohydrates, including pizza, toast, pasta, french fries, and even burgers (remember, burgers are inside buns!). Beer and other alcohol should also be avoided because they're high in carbohydrates too. Although most diets limit alcohol consumption because it's high in calories and offers little nutritional value, low carb diets particularly emphasize restricting them.

Despite the obvious restrictions, many foods can be enjoyed on a low carbohydrate diet. If you love meat you'll enjoy the opportunity to eat chicken, beef and other animal products. Low carb diets are extremely popular, as evidenced by the way they stay on the bestseller lists for such long periods of time. Low carb dieting is successful for many people, but it's a matter of finding a diet you can stay on because it suits you.

SIMPLE TIPS AND EXERCISE PLANS TO LOSE WEIGHT

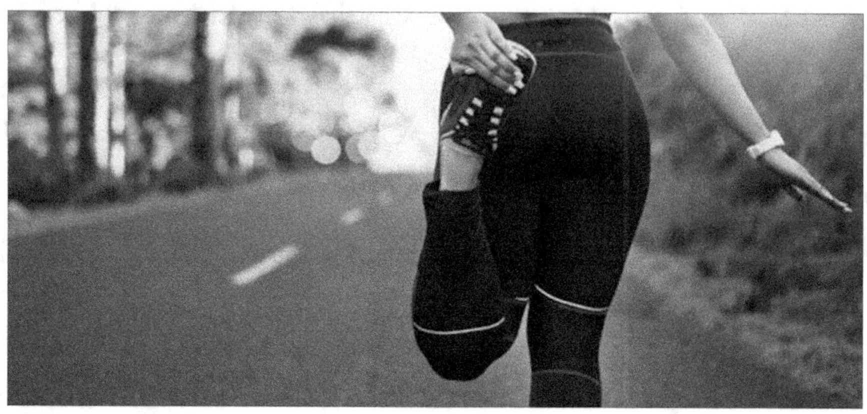

There are several ways to lose weight fast and melt away your fat instantly. However, most of them leave you unsatisfied as one realizes that shortcuts to lose weight are not sustainable in the long run. Weight loss is a combination of a well-formulated diet plan and a rigorous exercise regime. If you are wondering how to lose weight here are a few simple tips for weight loss and exercise plans to lose weight and reduce those inches:

1. Train your mind.

Weight loss is about a good diet, rigorous exercise regime but most importantly about mental conviction. Before starting out on a weight loss journey, mentally make a note of why you are taking this step and keep this reason to keep you going and prevent you from catering to those cravings by binge eating.

2. _Avoid food with high sugar content._

Insulin is the fat storage hormone in our bodies and sugary foods like desserts release insulin. This instantly raises our blood sugar level, in turn, resulting in fat storage. Lowering insulin also works as a detox for the body allowing kidneys to expel any excess sodium or nitrates, which may cause bloating. It's important to completely cut out fizzy drinks which also cause gas.

3. _Do not leave out a food group._

Every year the weight loss industry makes one or the other food group the worst for the body. It is best to have all fats, carbs, and proteins as part of our diet. Food rich in protein has been shown to boost one's metabolism and also reduces cravings

4. _Water is your savior._

Make sure to stay hydrated with water and other fluids throughout the day. One must drink at least 8 glasses of water a day to prevent all that bloating. A glass of water with lemon in it is recommended right after you wake up.

5. Fiber is key to a healthy gut.

Food like vegetables is high in fiber, which prevents constipation and also helps one get a flat belly soon. It also helps in better digestion and improving your immune system in the long run.

6. Stay away from fad diets.

The market today is flooded with diets like the GM diet, Atkins, Keto diet which all have very serious consequences to our bodies in the long run. Anything that comes fast, goes fast so remember to be patient and eat everything but in moderation.

Diet Plan for weight loss:

Here is a standard diet you can use for weight loss, before following any diet please consult a nutritionist/ dietitian. Everyone's body is unique, a single diet cannot be utilized by everyone.

- Breakfast: 3 egg whites OR Oatmeal with fruit and cup of green tea.

- Mid-morning snack: 150 gms of chicken cooked in vinegar and soy OR 1 steamed 6-inch corn tortilla with fresh or grilled vegetables (such as onions, green bell peppers, and tomatoes) and no-added-salt salsa.

- Lunch: Grilled fish with vegetables OR 2 Cups Mixed Greens with 1 Cup of Other Veggies, Chopped, Dressed with Aged Balsamic Vinegar

- Mid-afternoon snack: A salad of chickpeas OR a Banana and 1 Apple

- Dinner: Protein shake with any protein (Tofu, chicken, fish, etc) OR Salad with fresh ingredients.

Exercise plan to lose weight

Need some weight loss exercise? Follow an exercise plan that allows you to try a new thing daily. Engage in high cardio like running, Zumba, skipping but also hit the gym to lose weight. It is important to maintain muscle mass and it burns fat even after the workout is over. A great way to burn a good 1000 calories is a quick HIIT (High-Intensity Interval Training Workout) workout.

What is the Best Diet For Losing Weight and Fat?

We have all heard about those fad diets like the grapefruit diet or the apple diet. I am here to tell you diets that work. All of those diets are fad, crash, "stupid" diets. A real diet contains a mix of muscle building protein, energy filling carbs, and healthy fats for your heart.

For losing weight, ketosis is the best diet and is not a fad. In a keto diet, one would eat lots of protein and fats and little carbohydrates to get there body in a state of ketosis. Since there is no more glycogen in your body, from the lack of carbohydrates, your body will build ketone bodies from your fat tissues to fuel your body and your brain. As long as you are eating enough protein, you will preserve your muscle and lose pounds of fat easy.

Getting into ketosis takes about 3-7 days depending on your current glycogen storage. Ketosis feels odd at first because you will be lethargic and may experience headaches and even nausea. However, these symptoms go away. You will also drop lots of weight at first because of water weight.

Typical foods on a keto diet include nuts, whey protein, eggs, bacon, sausage, olive oil, butter, salmon, etc; anything that contains a high amount of protein and fats and no carbs. A vitamin pill is often taken in a keto diet since you can't eat many vegetables. (however, you can eat at least one bowl of salad)

It takes strong willpower to stay on keto because if you cheat once or eat something bad your body will be out of ketosis. A process that took 3-7 days now has to be re-done.

In short, Keto is the best short-term diet you can do for cutting.

FASTEST AND NATURAL WAY TO LOSE WEIGHT

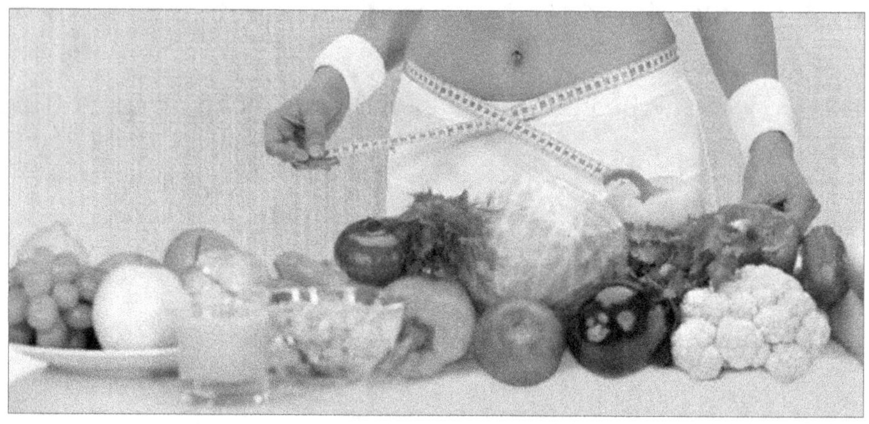

What is weight?

Weight loss is a major topic for discussion within and outside medical boundaries. In the medical arena, weight loss is seen as a method for gaining back one's health, while others are more concerned with the physical attributes that come about as a result of it, mainly in the form of better perceived physical appeal.

Why it is important to get rid of your extra body fat?

Generally, extra body fat indicates the presence of accumulated fatty substances that deposit themselves under the skin and hence show up easily. This extra body fat is largely believed to be an indication of ill-health, as it is a reflection of the fatty deposits that accumulate on the inner walls of arteries and arterioles, and it is of utmost importance to get rid of this body fat to get a healthy life with smart body

Facts regarding weight loss

Weight loss can be of two types, one which takes place unintentionally may be a result of illhealth. However, when it is a result of voluntary effort with the intention of improving one's health, it is a healthy process. Indeed, weight loss can be attained through different means; one may decide to exercise sufficiently to lose weight or resort to a change in diet or even a combination of the two. There are many people who resort to using medication to drop their weight rapidly. Medical practitioners dispute the merits of the latter, as the long-term effects of this measure are unpredictable.

Naturally, lose weight in a fun way

The best way to lose weight involves doing something as part of your routine that you enjoy. For some people, this involves having a few friends with whom they can go and visit a gymnasium regularly. Along with this, they might implement a diet that is sustainable and one that will take them towards good health and stay clear of wearing them thin on mineral resources and other important nutrients. Often, people fall for fad diets and they adhere to them along with an exercise routine, which is dangerous because in a short time they can find themselves depleting their vital resources.

Apart from using the gym, one may decide on playing a sport one fancies. Some people are known to begin with mild to medium intensity training in martial arts, depending on their age, state of health, etc.

It is important to remember that when taking up a physical activity that suits you in the long run, you need to have a balanced diet and stay clear of medication to lose weight. If you decide to use medication, you might lose weight rapidly, but when you take yourself off it, you might experience weight gain, dissatisfaction, and lethargy amid other side effects.

Is it good to use pills to lose weight?

While pills may have tremendous effects when it comes to a rapid loss in weight, there are medical concerns. First of all, it is not a natural way of losing weight, which means that it does not change a human being's habit. In turn, when a person stops using these pills, they may start gaining weight again because they have not changed their lifestyles. Additionally, medical experts believe there could be long-term consequences when people use pills to lose weight. The ultimate result of using pills to lose weight has not been defined, which seriously means that there might be severe risks associated with their use.

Methods to reduce your weight quickly

While long-term and sustainable implementation of diets along with appropriate physical activity is recommended for losing weight, sometimes people want to lose weight rapidly. This is particularly the case when they face serious health and life-threatening issues.

1. One method of losing weight rapidly includes using pills. One has to undergo an assessment prior to using this method. Only a physician who has examined an individual can recommend these. The results are

startling, as people are known to start showing signs of weight loss in a matter of days.

2 . Another method of losing weight, although a little slower, is through diets that subtract your weight gaining substances. An example of such a diet is the Cabbage Diet. These kinds of diets have to be administered over a short period, as long-term adherence to it could ruin your health.

3 . Apart from adjusting what one consumes in order to lose weight, there is also the concept of intense exercise routines that people can put them self's through. This helps one to lose weight due to the fact that calories get burned rapidly. One example of a typical exercise in this method is the treadmill. The more you use, the more you will lose weight. However, here again, there is an issue of sustainability, as the intensity of exercise is sure to wear a person out after a short amount of time.

4 . Another method of losing weight rapidly that does not work for all people is by skipping meals. Many people decide to skip lunch or dinner in order to cut down on around onethird of their consumption. While some people are known to experience weight loss through this approach, medical experts ponder over the wisdom of it. This is because there can be severe issues with one's digestive system when meals are skipped; digestive

fluids begin to act on the very walls of the digestive tract that produce them.

Tips to help you lose weight:

It is important to keep in mind that people of all ages are likely to suffer from overweight-related health issues. However, the following points pertain to people between the ages of 20 and 40.

- People are known to use weight loss pills and other formulas for losing weight. These are not really advised unless you feel that you are running out of time and need to lose weight rapidly before something severe happens to you. Using pills and medication for weight loss does not form any good habits, and you are likely to go back t your old bad routine and eating habits.

- People past the age of 20 are known to suffer from a condition known as obesity. They may be suffering from this due to sustained childhood obesity. Since this issue is most likely to have been prompted by inactivity, it is thought the individual has to be gradually drawn into a healthier lifestyle.

- Whether you have been overweight since your childhood or not, you still have to get into a healthier mode of physical activity. Initially, one can start by taking leisurely strolls in the mornings. The length and sped of these can be gradually be increased in order to boost the burning of calories.

- Intense and strenuous workouts are also used in order to burn calories. However, this needs to be implemented in accordance with...

- Consuming naturally produced foods that are meant to reduce weight through their medicinal properties. This includes the consumption of things like Green Tea that is known to cut your cut. Some people prefer to go for consuming grapefruit juice. This is known to be very effective, but they need to discuss this with their physician, especially if they are on medication.

- Non-sustainable diets such as fad diets can be used for reducing one's weight. The weight loss may be rapid, but the diet itself may not be sustainable.

- Sustainable diets are those that are well balanced and don't deny you of your vital nutrients. These diets tend to show slower progress, but in the long run, they can lead you to better eating habits and a better lifestyle.

- Sustainable diets and adequate exercise is thought to be the right approach to losing weight. The intensity of the exercise may vary according to one's age and physical well being, and the diet too can be adjusted to meet the nutritional demands of an individual.

Weight Loss is All in Your Mind

It's often the will to do something that leads you to success. Indeed, many people end up remaining unhealthy and fat throughout their lives because they simply believe that they can't lose weight. This is completely contrary to the truth! If you develop the will and have every intention of losing weight, you can say that you have already won half the battle. Indeed, it is the will to achieve the goal that will drive you, and one may even go as far as saying that it's all about how much you really want to lose weight, gain your good health back and also look great.

Natural Weight Loss and Fat Burning Advice to Change Your Life

Consuming the right foods in the right proportion can help you lose weight. Such a diet has to be designed carefully by a dietician. Along with this, you will need to have a decent exercise routine in order to guarantee a healthy routine. The right activity along with the right consumption of food goes hand-in-hand. Over a period of time, when you adhere to this lifestyle, you are bound to experience the merits of it.

The best way to lose weight is through a natural process that includes adequate exercise that burns calories coupled with a decent diet that reduces the unnecessary weight gaining and fatty substances that ruin our health. If one succeeds in putting these two together, it is almost certain that you will lose weight and settle into a healthy lifestyle.

FAST WEIGHT LOSS
IN 12 EASY STEPS

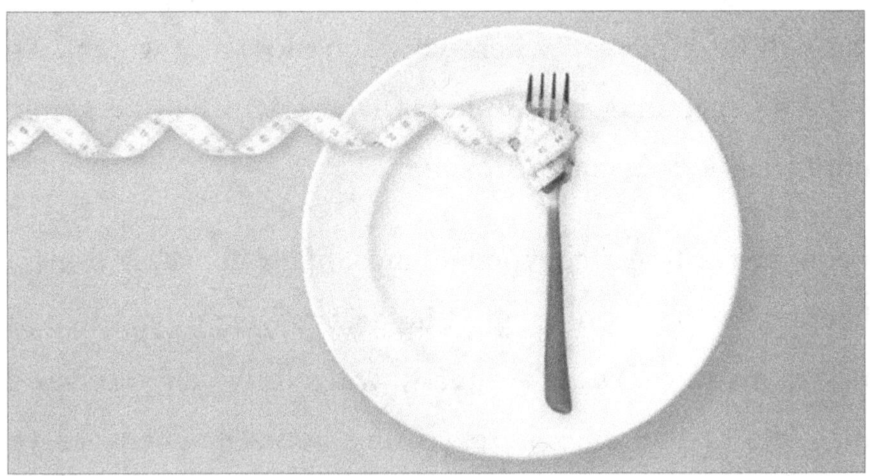

You can experience fast weight loss in 12 easy steps. Many of my patients and friends lost weight fast, shedding 1 to 2 pounds every week without following some crazy fad diet or taking a dangerous diet pill. Just 12 easy steps to lose weight and keep it off!

Let's get to it...

It's the dream of an overweight person to lose weight. The unfortunate thing is that very few people know the right things to do to lose weight safely. To help you out, here are 12 tips to losing weight safely:

Seek Motivation

Let nobody lie to you that it's easy to lose weight. Sometimes you will hit a plateau where you don't lose any weight. You will also encounter some phases where you will be gaining more weight than you are losing.

If you are faint-hearted, you will most likely give up. To ensure that you keep on pursuing your dream weight, you need to seek motivation. There are many ways in which you can do this. One of the ways is rewarding yourself whenever you make progress. You should also surround yourself with people who are also interested in losing weight.

Don't Skip Meals

While you should cut on the number of calories that you consume, you shouldn't starve your body. Many people make the mistake of skipping meals in order to reduce the calories that they consume. You should note that when you skip meals, you provoke your body to get into starvation mode thus you have the tendency of experiencing weight gain.

Instead of skipping meals, you should divide your meals into small. To avoid starvation you should take 4-6 small meals a day.

Reduce Sodium Consumption

Sodium causes water retention which causes the weight to stay on your body. To lose weight you should stay away from high sodium foods. As a rule of thumb, you should stay away from convenience foods as they are usually full of sodium.

Eat Right

The food that you eat is of great importance. As a rule of thumb, you should avoid foods that have a lot of calories. The best way of avoiding unhealthy foods is ensuring that you prepare the food in your home.

You should also be cautious of the food labels. Before you buy any food, ensure that you have thoroughly gone through the labels and ensure that all the ingredients are in their right proportions.

Exercise

Exercises play a major role in weight loss. They not only increase your rate of metabolism, but they also aid in burning fat. Experts recommend that you should engage in 30 minutes to 1-hour exercises for three days a week. For ideal results, you should engage in both cardio and strength building exercises.

Set Realistic Goals

It's good to be ambitious; however, you shouldn't be too ambitious. Although you might be interested in losing weight, you shouldn't expect to lose all the weight within a few days you should allow the process to be gradual. For example, you should aim at losing 1-2 pounds a day. Aiming to lose more weight than this is not only unhealthy, it's also unachievable thus you end up giving up.

1. Eat 250 Fewer Calories a Day

Cutting out 250 calories is not hard. Cut your bread servings in half, substitute starches with vegetables, and stop eating process sugars and foods.

2. Burn 250 Calories a Day

Water aerobics, walking with calisthenics, biking, rowing, stair steps, and jogging for 30 minutes will do the trick.

3. Block Carbohydrate Absorption

Excess calories from carbohydrates end up as body fat. Taking 800 mg/day of white kidney bean extract and 125 mg/day each of two brown seaweed kelp, bladderwrack, and Ascophyllum, will turn off the enzymes responsible for carbohydrate absorption.

4. Block Fat Absorption

The lipase enzyme is responsible for fat absorption. Block it with a prescription drug called Orlistat (Alli is the over-the-counter version). Take 5 grams of a soluble fiber supplement 15 to 30 minutes before each major meal for additional help.

5. Break Leptin Resistance

Leptin is a hormone that tells your brain to stop eating. But as we age, leptin has difficulty getting to the brain...this is called leptin resistance. Take

300 mg/day of Irvingia gabonensis, a West African plant that breaks leptin resistance.

6. Restore Your Resting Metabolic Rate

Burn more calories at rest by supplementing with 500 mg/day of green tea extract and 100 mg/day of 7-keto-DHEA.

That's it. Fast weight loss in 6 easy steps.

These are tips on how to lose weight. For ideal results, you should avoid shady programs that promise to help you lose all of the extra weight in one or two weeks. Always remember that fast weight loss isn't healthy. It's also neither permanent.

LOW CARB DIET WEIGHT LOSS– IS THE LOW CARB DIET MORE SUITABLE FOR THE OBESE?

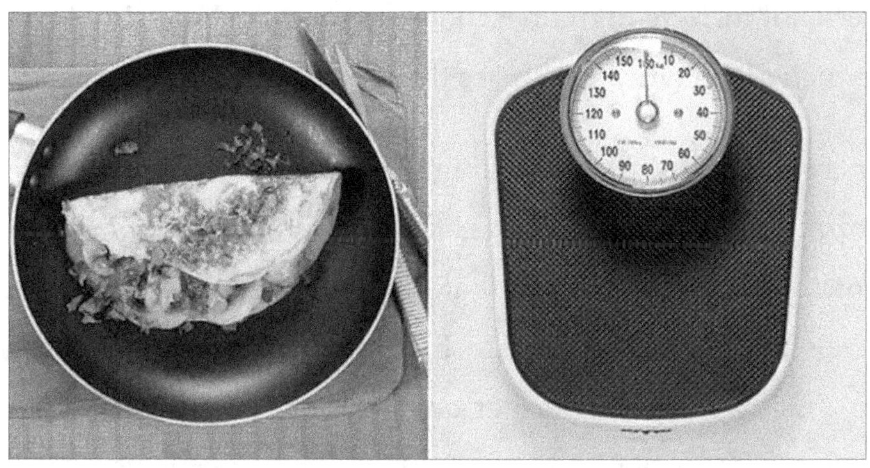

There is a countless number of different diets that people can use to lose weight. The truth is that most of them are junk and don't work at all. So choosing the right kind of diet that helps you lose weight and more importantly keep it off, is essential. Although low carb diets are certainly not suitable for everyone, if you are seriously overweight and have over 50 pounds to lose, then a low carb diet might work very well for you.

Low carb diet weight loss

We all know that carbohydrates provide energy for the body and if they are in excess, like everything else, then they will be stored as fat. It is also clear that a high carbohydrate intake, that does not include high fiber foods but does include simple and refined carbohydrates, causes the chronic release of insulin.

A chronic insulin level inhibits hormone sensitive lipase, the enzyme that behaves like a gatekeeper allowing fatty acids to flow out of the fat cells. But at the same time elevated insulin levels also kick up levels of lipoprotein lipase another such enzyme that has gatekeeper qualities. And these gatekeepers welcome fatty acids into your fat cells, making you fatter. Insulin is also an appetite stimulant and it increases the cravings for food. This fat storing and appetite stimulating effect is magnified by heavier individuals. Research has shown that an obese person, eating 40 grams of carbs, will secrete more insulin than a lean person, eating the same amount of carbs.

By reducing carbohydrates and increasing protein levels in the diet, means that your body has to spend a lot more energy to break down protein than carbohydrates. The more energy your body has to spend to break down protein means the more calories you burn. Of course, the danger of very low carb diets is the lack of energy since we get most of our energy from carbohydrates. So staying on a very low carbohydrate diet for long periods, is really impossible. Never go too far with low carb diets.

HOW TO FIND YOUR MOTIVATION TO LOSE WEIGHT HEALTHILY AND NATURALLY

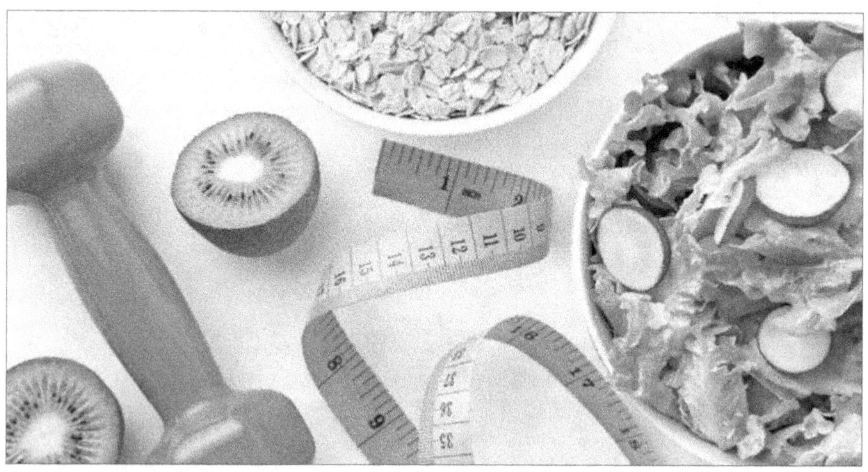

When we want to change our bodies, the obvious solution is to simply start exercising or take up a new hobby or play sports. This is the solution to the problem, but before these events take place, the mental block that is motivation rears its ugly head.

Motivation is basically the driver behind why we will and won't do certain things in our life. We have to find some way of pushing ourselves to do the things that we need to do to get to where we want to get to.

Everyone has different levels of motivation for different things, and it really comes down to what the person values more in their life.

Now in regards to motivation for weight loss, this issue has to be addressed correctly otherwise things can be affected in the long term.

When you first decide that you want to lose weight, there has to be some kind of motivational reason behind this decision. There could be any number of reasons why you want to lose weight, they could be personal or family reasons or even peer pressure.

Many people will really struggle with this hurdle, as they are not doing what they want for the correct reasons. If you decided that you want to lose weight, because you are so unhappy with your body, and you won't feel better about yourself, then you this is your motivation to lose weight.

There is a real purpose for the reason, and when you have a purpose for a decision, the actions you take are normally more much focused and decisive.

Let's take the other scenario that you want to lose weight for a family member, then this reason is a fairly strong reason to lose weight, but it is not going to motivate you as hard as doing it for yourself would be.

Now to find motivation, this can come from many different places. One of the best ways to find motivation is to buddy up with a friend who wants to reach the same goals as you and you both motivate and spur each other on to lose weight. This can work really well because you feed off each other's energy.

Another great way to get motivated is to set a date to reach a goal by. When you set a date you set yourself a challenge, by doing this you will become more motivated to reach the goal. A good way to bring this up, even more, is to give yourself an incentive to reach the goal, this will also help you with motivation.

The next strategy to help you find motivation is to make sure that you are going into a new challenge with a clear mind, with no bad obstacles that can cause a hindrance to your progress. Motivation is very hard to find and keep when your life is run down with financial stress, health issues, and family problems.

A common mistake that people make when they want to lose weight is that they put pictures/posters of size zero models on the walls in their houses. The idea here is that you will become more inspired to reach the desired figure in the posters, but that opposite is actually true according to extensive research.

The reason why this theory is less effective for motivation is that people are more likely to become discouraged by creating unrealistic self-standards. This will then cause a lack of motivation and the person will most likely give in on reaching their ideal body shape from the poster.

Another common reason why people lose motivation to lose weight is that they focus too much on the numbers. When you have decided that you want to lose say 10lbs within 2 months, all of your energy and focus is centered on this one goal, and if you do not reach it, you will feel bad and most likely lose motivation. This should be avoided.

Another reason why people lose motivation when they are trying to lose weight is that they do not have a plan of action in place from the start. A weight loss goal or program should be treated like a business plan and specific details should be written down and put on paper to help the individual stay motivated.

When creating a plan of action to lose weight, there need to be a few factors tailored into the plan, realistic, measurable and free from any in-effective strategies. If you have an unrealistic plan of action for your goals from the start, you will lose motivation very quickly and most likely give in on the goals that you want to reach.

A very useful way to stay motivated towards your weight loss goals is to give yourself rewards every so often when you have reached a certain milestone. A good way to do it by starting off with small incentives or small prizes and makes the prizes bigger as you reach your ultimate goal. This practice is often overlooked but very powerful as you have something to work towards each time, this provides a new lease for motivation.

SWEET AFTERNOON MADE HEALTHIER WITH LOW CARB BREAD PUDDING AND OTHER SNACKS

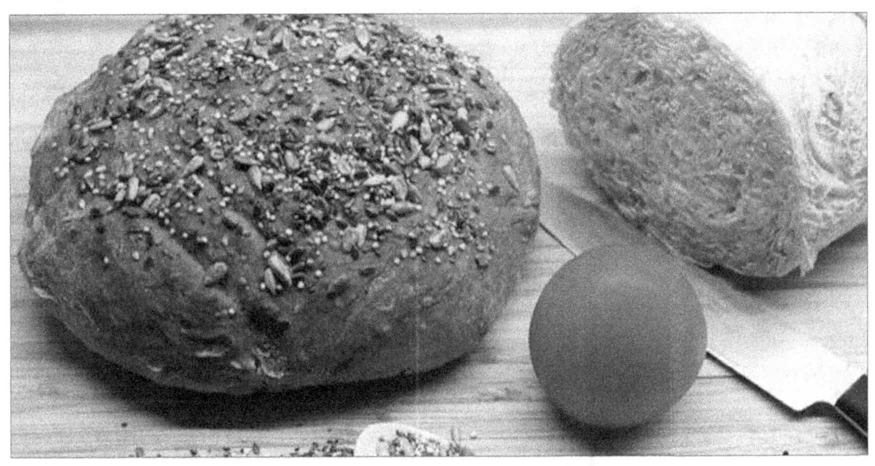

You start the day with a well balanced, healthy breakfast and follow it with a nutritious lunch, happy to be eating right and feeling great thanks to it. But by the late afternoon, you're done waiting for dinner and you reach for a quick dessert, telling yourself that a couple of pieces of chocolate or a cookie won't do any harm. Unfortunately, more often than not it doesn't end on just two little pieces of dark chocolate or one oatmeal cookie, and what was supposed to be a little snack before a healthy dinner turns into a whole sweet meal in itself. A sweet dinner every once in a while is not bad, it will help with your cravings, as long as you skip the bag of mini chocolate candy bars or a batch of rich brownies and go for treats that are better for you.

For a warm and fruity dessert in place for dinner try some delicious bread pudding. However, make it with low carb bread, add rich spices like ground ginger, cinnamon, and real vanilla, mix in your favorite fruit, like apples, cranberries or raisins. When serving, stop short of pouring rich sauce on it or decorating it with heaps of whipped cream, and instead sprinkle a dash of spices and maybe drizzle just a bit of real maple syrup or honey on top. If you eat your bread pudding still warm, the richness of the flavor and the different textures will make it so tasty in and of itself that you won't be missing any calorie-rich additions.

If you like the idea of a warm and fruity dessert but are not too fond of it being bread or dough based, your best bet is to light up your grill. Stick your favorite fruit cut up into chunks onto skewers and place on the grill, or if you don't have one, on a cast iron pan or in the oven and keep it just long enough to get the grill marks. Fruit prepared this way will taste great, and you can bring more flavor out by adding some nutty spices and serving it with fresh mint leaves on top. For a more filling dish prepare a yogurt dip using a thick, Greek, natural yogurt and mixing it with spices, honey or just the softened fruit.

Some people like their snack soft and gooey, others prefer a bit of crunch. If you like to bite into something crispy, consider making pita bread chips by cutting your pita into triangles and tossing it in the oven or skillet until they harden, and preparing a selection of delicious dips to go with them. A smooth fruit and yogurt dip, a thick guacamole on a sweet side, homemade peanut or almond butter, spicy apple sauce or a banana cream cheese are just some of the dips that will go great with your chips, and the great thing is that if you have any left over, you can always grab them the next day for lunch.

Chocolate, candy, cookies, ice cream and all kinds of other sweets are delicious, but if eaten too often they can lead to weight and health issues. That's why if you do have a sweet tooth, turning to more health-conscious sweet snacks is a must, and if you let your imagination run wild, those good for you snacks will be as delicious as they are sweet.

LOW CARB BREAD
AFTER A WORKOUT?

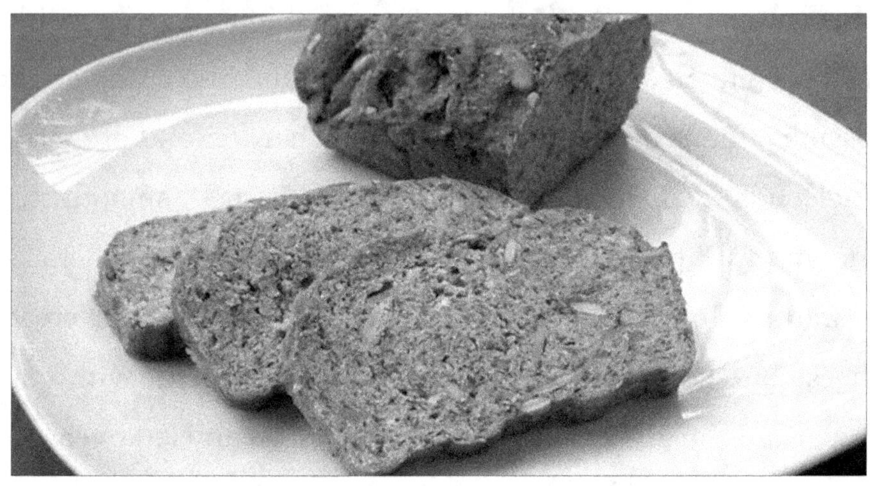

Whether you exercise to lose weight or to improve your heart health, whether you love it or treat it as a necessary unpleasant duty towards your body, whether it's a daily routine or something you do once a week, you probably know to not eat too close before you start your workout and to hydrate throughout. What you may not know, though, is that after you're done your body needs some nourishment to aid post-exercise recovery and to keep you in that hard-earned good shape.

After a good workout, your priority needs to be repairing muscle tissue and replenishing glycogen stores, and that means a combination of protein with often dreaded carbohydrates. Even if your typical menu choices limit carbs and you prefer to reach for low carb bread, plain vegetables and fruit or cottage cheese to do that, after strenuous workout carbs are not only allowed, they are beneficial.

If you have sweet tooth, peanut butter is a great item to munch on. You can spread it over a rice cake and top it with a banana, you can dip apple chunks in it or you can make peanut butter and unsweetened jelly sandwich on whole wheat bread or English muffin. Either one of these choices will satisfy both your sweet tooth and your need for post-workout nutrition. And if you love your snacks sweet but don't like or can't eat peanut butter, you should reach for some natural yogurt mixed with delicious berries, you can make a protein shake with banana or munch on a mix of dried fruit and nuts. For a great crunch with just a bit of sweet to it, a high fiber, low sugar cereal with skim milk is a perfect snack that will satisfy you easily after your workout.

For those looking for savory flavors after exercising, a turkey sandwich on whole wheat bread, with some avocado and lettuce, pita bread with cheese and crackers are quick and satisfying.

And if you have some time and get home quickly after finishing your exercise, a veggie-loaded omelet, stir fry with some chicken for lean protein or pancakes and eggs without the butter and syrup but with a serving of fresh fruit on the side will take care of all your needs post-workout. Just be sure to chase whatever you eat with some water, and your body will feel good enough to head to work if you exercise in the morning or just right to wind down with the family if you work out later in the day.

GET THE FACTS ON LOW CARB BREAD RECIPE IDEAS

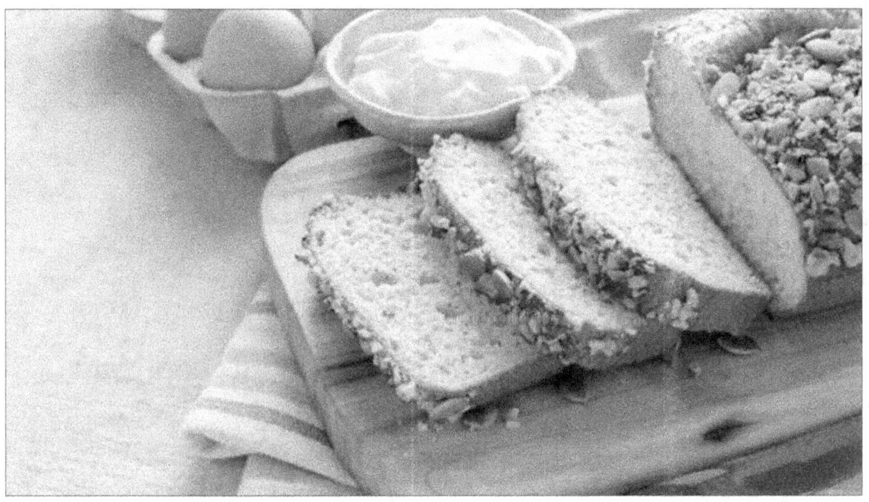

If you are a bread fan but you need to reduce the carbohydrate that you often eat from bread, low carb bread recipe is your excellent option. Bread can be included in your diet menu as long as you select the best low carb bread recipe.

As a matter of fact, there are some great options starts from a low carb cheesecake recipe to a low carb apple muffins recipe that you can include in your recipe book.

Cook Your Own Bread

In order to be able to take in bread to your diet, there are actually plenty of recipes ideas that you may want to practice. Simply the bread is one of the much-loved bread recipe ideas that you can try.

For this recipe, all you need are a number of ingredients that include 1/2 cup cream, 1 large egg, 1/2 cup warm water, 1 tablespoon oil, 1 cup gluten flour, 1 cup oat flour, ¼ teaspoon salt, 1 tablespoon sugar and 2 tablespoons yeast.

A bread machine is what you'll need, and you simply put in the ingredients into the machine in the array given.

Afterward, bake the bread at 375°F for thirty minutes. Cheddar cheese bread is another more innovative recipe you may want to try. This recipe will take only about a half hour to prepare.

For it, you'll need 1/3 cup soy protein, 1/3 cup soy flour, 2 large eggs, and 1/2 teaspoon baking powder.

Other ingredients that you want to have are 1/2 cup cedar cheese, 2 tablespoons sour cream, 2 teaspoons oregano, and grated 2 tablespoons olive oil.

How to Make a Low Carb Bread at Home

The sedentary lifestyle of today's world has increased the demand for low carb and fat-free diets to maintain good health and avoid problems such as high blood pressure, diabetes, and obesity. Low carb diets are also known to help overcome fatigue caused due to increased insulin levels in the blood. If you make low carb diets a part of your life you will feel increased levels of energy, lesser cravings for sweets and improved dental hygiene. Since bread machine recipes are the most staple part of any diet it is, therefore, important to substitute regular bread with low carb bread.

The good news is that you can prepare it at home in a few easy steps. Here is a low carb bread machine recipe for you to try out.

What you will need:

- Dry yeast (bread machine) - 1 packet

- Sugar - 1/2 teaspoon

- Warm water - 1 1/8 cups (at about 100F)

- Olive oil - 3 tablespoons

- Baking powder - 1 1/2 teaspoons

- Salt - 1 teaspoon

- Splenda - 1 tablespoon

- Gluten-free wheat flour - 1 cup

- Oat flour - 1/4 cup

- Soy flour - 3/4 cup

- Flaxseed meal - 1/4 cup

- Unprocessed wheat barn - 1/4 cup **Directions:**

- The recipe is for simple bread cycle but if your bread machine instructions call for a different setting for gluten-free flour you must use that cycle.

- Clean the bread machine pan and dry it thoroughly before using.

- Open the packet of yeast and put the contents in the bread pan.

- Add the water and sugar and stir to mix.

- Let it rest for some time to let the yeast ferment.

- In the meantime, mix the dry ingredients in a bowl.

- Pour the olive oil in the machine pan and add the dry ingredients on top of it.

- Set the machine to run on the basic cycle and let it cook for 3-4 hours.

- Cool in the pan for some time before removing from the pan and cooling on a wire rack.

- Cut in slices to serve.

Tips:

- You can add rye flour in place of soy and oat flour if you like the taste.

- You can also add sunflower seeds or sesame seeds in place of flax seeds.

- The small amount of sugar does not add to any extra calories as it is only used for the activation of the yeast.

- This bread can be stored in the fridge for up to 2 weeks.

- You can use it in any bread dishes as normal bread such as a sandwich wrapper, toast, or simple bread and butter.

- This bread also makes a great base for homemade pizza.

EASY KETO RECIPES

1. BAKED PESTO CHICKEN RECIPE

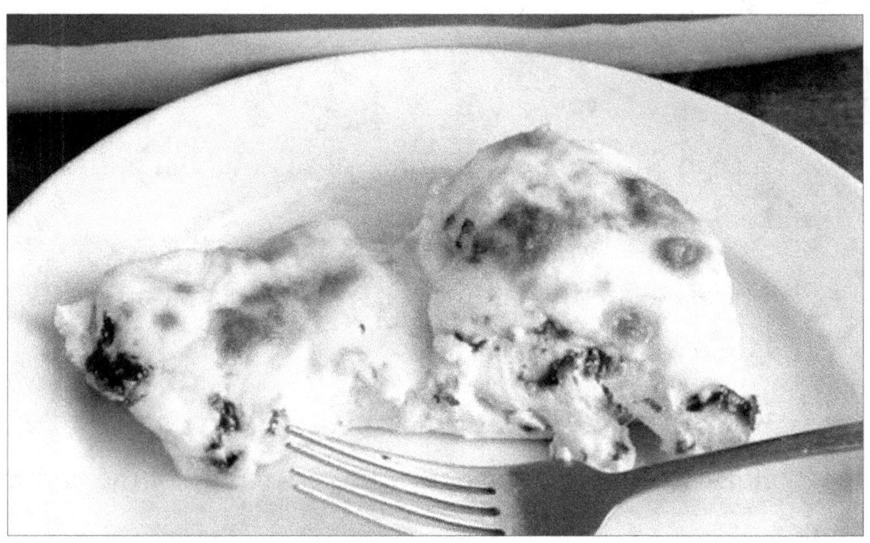

Prep Time: 5 mins, Cook Time: 35 minsm, Total Time: 40 mins

Servings: 4

Ingredients

- 4 chicken breasts about 1.5 lb, sliced in half widthwise to make 8 pieces

- 3 tbsp basil pesto

- 8 oz mozzarella thinly sliced or shredded

- 1/2 tsp salt

- 1/4 tsp black pepper

<u>Directions:</u>

- Preheat oven to 350.

- Spray baking dish with cooking spray. Place chicken in the bottom in a single layer and sprinkle with the salt and pepper. Spread the pesto on the chicken. Put the mozzarella on top.

- Bake for 35-45 minutes until the chicken is 160 degrees and the cheese is golden and bubbly. You can broil it for a few minutes at the end to brown the cheese if you want.

2 . EASY KETO CHICKEN SALAD RECIPE

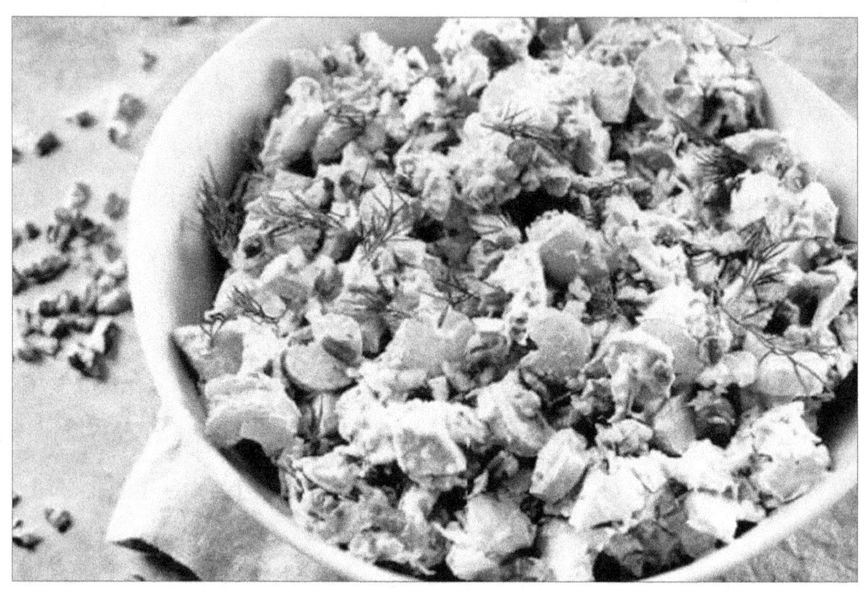

Cook Time: 15 mins

Total Time: 1 hr 30 mins

Servings: 6

<u>Ingredients</u>

- 1.5 lb chicken breast

- 3 ribs celery, diced

- 1/2 cup mayo

- 2 tsp brown mustard

- 1/2 tsp pink Himalayan salt

- 2 tbsp fresh dill, chopped

- 1/4 cup chopped pecans

Directions:

1. Preheat oven to 450 degrees and line baking sheet with parchment paper.

2. Bake chicken breast until cooked throughout, about 15 minutes.

3. Remove chicken from oven and allow to cool. After completely cooled, cut chicken into bite-sized pieces.

4. In a large bowl, add chicken, celery, mayo, brown mustard, and salt. Toss until chicken is fully coated and ingredients are well-combined.

5. Cover the bowl with lid or plastic wrap and refrigerate until chilled, about 1-2 hours.

6. When ready to serve, add fresh dill and chopped pecans and lightly toss. Serve chilled and enjoy!

3. SPINACH-MOZZARELLA STUFFED BURGERS RECIPE

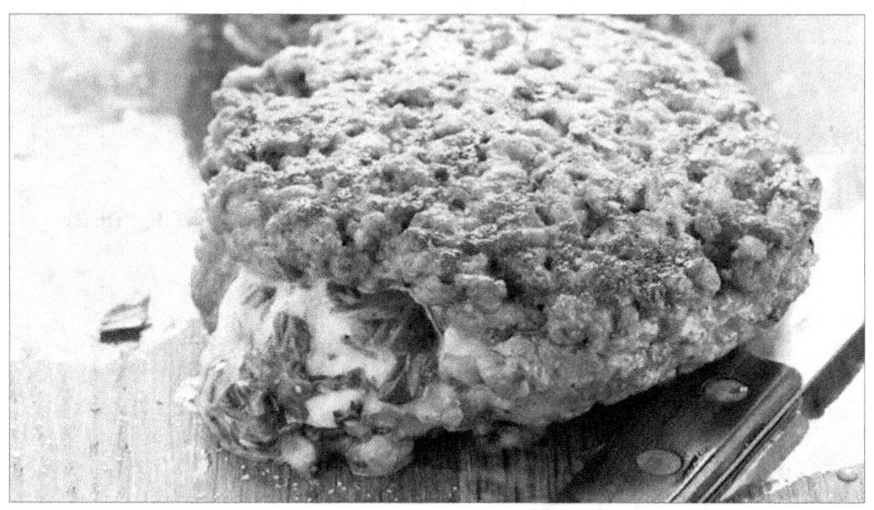

- Prep Time: 15 mins

- Cook Time: 10 mins

- Total Time: 25 mins

Servings: 4

Ingredients

- 1½ lbs ground chuck

- teaspoon salt

- ¾ teaspoon ground black pepper

- cups fresh spinach, firmly packed

- ½ cup shredded mozzarella cheese (about 4 oz)

- 2 tablespoons grated Parmesan cheese

Directions:

1. In a medium bowl, combine ground beef, salt, and pepper.

2. Scoop about 1/3 cup of mixture and with dampened hands shape into 8 patties about ½inch thick. Place in the refrigerator.

3. Place spinach in a saucepan over medium-high heat. Cover and cook for 2 minutes, until wilted.

4. Drain and let cool. With your hands squeeze the spinach to extract as much liquid as possible.

5. Transfer to a cutting board, chop the spinach and place in a bowl.

6. Stir in mozzarella cheese and Parmesan.

7. Scoop about ¼ cup of stuffing and mound in the center of 4 patties,

8. Cover with remaining 4 patties, and seal the edges by pressing firmly together.

9 . Cut each patty with your hands to round out the edges, and press on the top to flatten slightly into a single thick patty.

1 0 . Heat a grill or a grill pan to medium-high (if you're using an outdoor grill lightly oil the grill grates).

1 1 . Grill burgers for 5 to 6 minutes on each side.

1 2 . Serve!

4. KETO BRUNCH SPREAD RECIPE

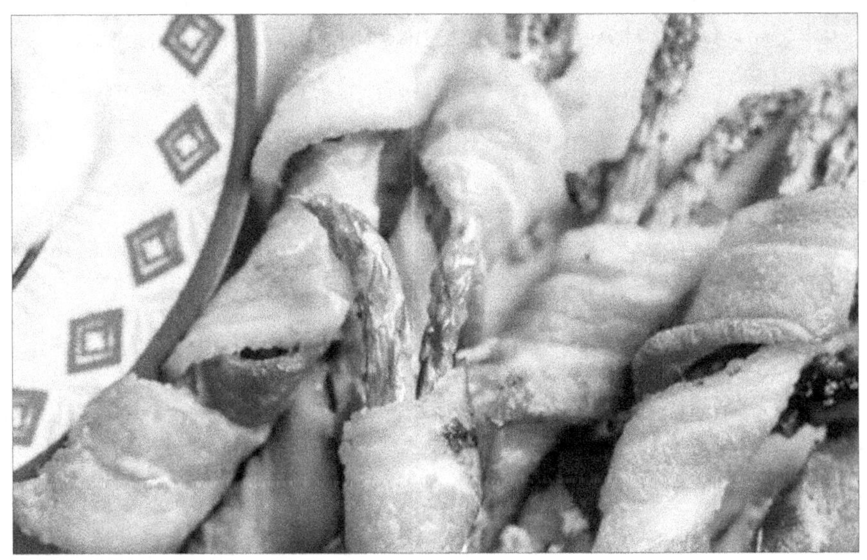

Prep Time: 10 mins Cook Time: 20 mins Total Time: 30 mins

Servings: 4

Ingredients

- 4 large eggs

- 24 asparagus spears

- 12 slices of pastured, sugar-free bacon

Directions:

1. Pre-heat your oven to 400F.

2. Trim your asparagus about an inch from the bottoms. Then in pairs, wrap them with one slice of bacon. Hold your spears firmly and close together with one hand as you wind the slice of bacon starting from the bottom, to the top of the spear. Gently pull the bacon as you wind it, so it wraps tightly. Place it on a sheet pan.

3. Repeat with the remaining asparagus, so you have 12 pairs wrapped in bacon.

4. Place in the oven set the timer for 20 minutes.

5. In this time, bring a small pot of water to a rapid boil. Gently place 4 large eggs in the boiling water. Set another time for 6 minutes.

6. Prepare a bowl with ice water. When the 6 minutes are up, use a slotted spoon or tongs to quickly transfer your eggs to the ice bath. Let them sit for 2 minutes before peeling the tops off.

7. Gently crack the top of the egg on a hard surface and peel away the shell to reveal the tip of the egg.

8. When the asparagus is ready, serve on a tray or cutting board. If you don't have an egg holder use espresso cups to hold your eggs up.

9. With a small spoon scoop out the tops of the soft boiled eggs to reveal a perfectly runny yolk.

10. Dip your asparagus spears into your eggs. Feast, enjoy!

5. SPICY KETO CHEESE CRISPS RECIPE

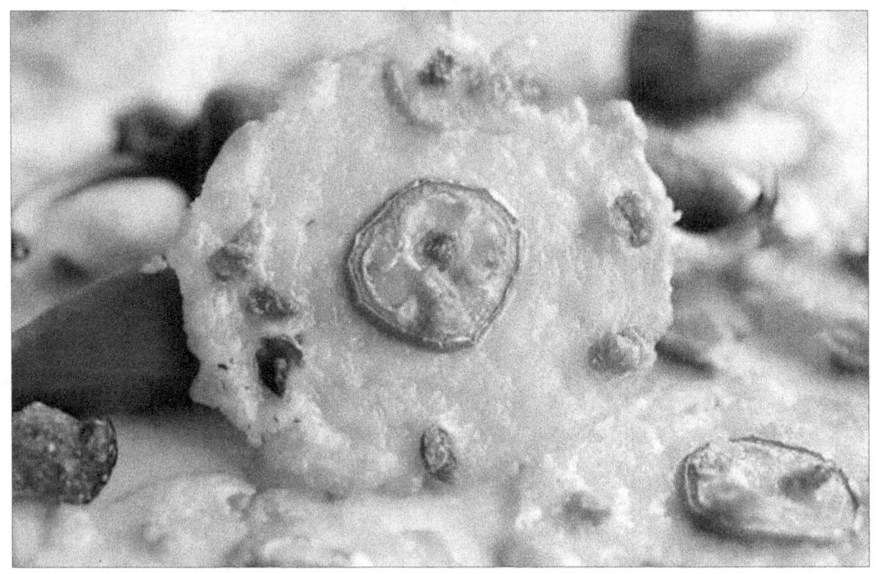

Prep Time: 5 mins Cook Time: 10 mins Total Time: 15 mins

Servings: 12

<u>Ingredients</u>

- Grass-fed cheddar cheese

- medium-sized jalapeno

- slices of bacon

<u>Directions:</u>

1. Preheat oven to 425 degrees and line a baking sheet with parchment paper or a Silpat.

2. Add even heaped tablespoons of cheese to the prepared baking sheet. Place one slice of jalapeño in the center of the mound. Sprinkle with crumbled bacon.

3. Bake on high for 7-10 minutes until cheese is melted and edges are browned.

4. Remove from oven and let cool completely until crisp.

6. PERFECT KETO AVOCADO BREAKFAST BOWL RECIPE

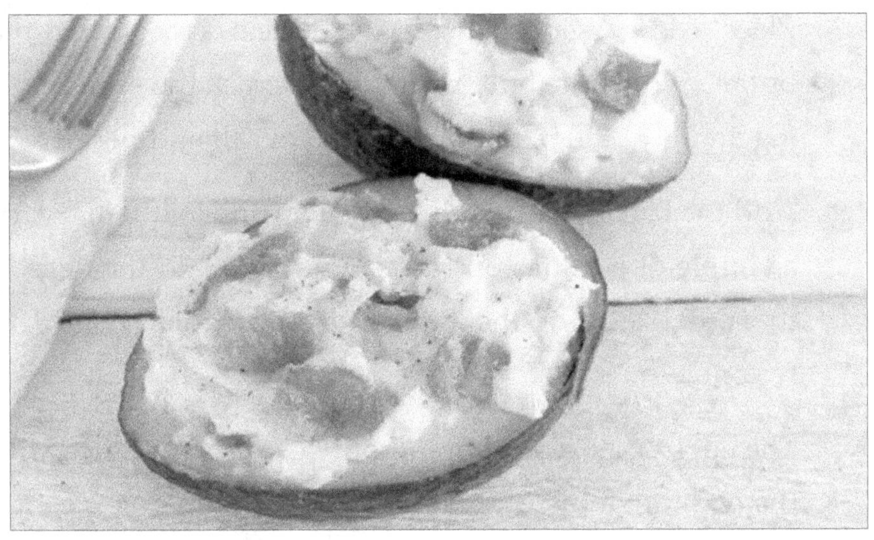

Prep Time: 5 mins Cook Time: 15 mins Total Time: 20 mins

Servings: 1

Ingredients

- 1 avocado, halved and the stone removed

- 1 tbsp salted butter

- 3 large free range eggs

- 3 rashers of bacon, cut into small pieces Pinch of salt and black pepper

Directions:

1. Start off by scooping out most of the avocado flesh, leaving about a ½ inch around the avocado.

2. Place a large saucepan on a low heat and add in the butter. Whilst the butter is melting, crack the eggs into a jug and beat them, adding a pinch of salt and pepper.

3. Add the bacon to one side of the pan and let them fry for a couple of minutes on their own. Then add the eggs to the other side of the pan and stir regularly as they scramble.

4. The eggs and bacon should both be done 5 minutes after the eggs are added to the pan. If you find your eggs are done a little before the bacon, remove the scrambled eggs from the pan and place in a bowl.

5. Mix the bacon pieces and scrambled eggs together in a bowl, then spoon into the avocado bowls and get to eatin'!

7. MEAT-LOVER PIZZA CUPS RECIPE

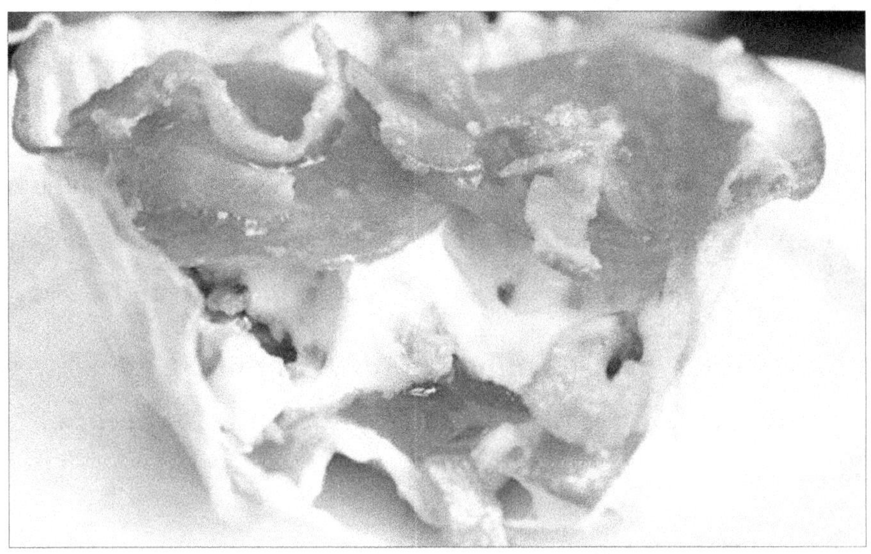

Prep Time: 15 mins Cook Time: 11 mins Total Time: 26 mins

Servings: 12

Ingredients

- 12 deli ham slices

- 1 lb. bulk Italian sausage

- 12 Tbsp sugar-free pizza sauce

- 3 cups grated mozzarella cheese

- 24 pepperoni slices

- 1 cup cooked and crumbled bacon

<u>Directions:</u>

1. Preheat oven to 375 F. Brown Italian sausage in a frying pan, draining excess grease.

2. Line 12-cup muffin tin with ham slices. Divide sausage, pizza sauce, mozzarella cheese, pepperoni slices, and bacon crumbles between each cup, in that order.

3. Bake at 375 for 10 minutes. Broil for 1 minute until cheese bubbles and browns and the edges of the meat toppings look crispy.

4. Remove pizza cups from muffin tin and set on a paper towel to prevent the bottoms from getting wet. Enjoy immediately or refrigerate and reheat in toaster oven or microwave.

8. CHICKEN CAESAR RECIPE

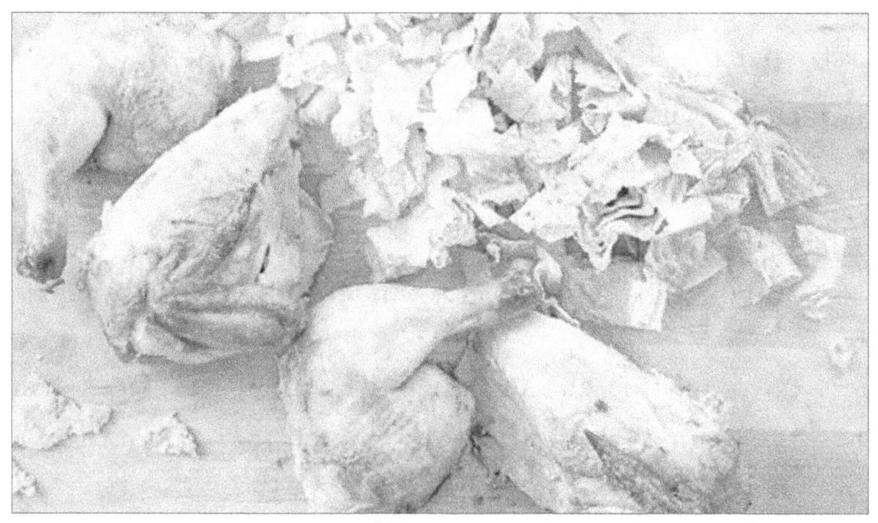

Prep Time: 48 hrs 5 mins Cook Time: 1 hr 25 mins Total Time: 49 hrs 30 mins

Servings: 6

Ingredients

- 1 Whole Pastured Chicken (4-5lbs)

- 1 cup Caesar salad dressing (for a dairy-free option, we recommend Tessamae's) Sea Salt

- 1/4 cup olive oil

- 5-6 Romaine Hearts

- 12+ Parmesan Crisps

Directions:

First, spatchcock your chicken. This will make it easier to marinate and it will cook faster and more evenly. Do this by using kitchen shears and cutting alongside the vertebrae on both sides. Remove the vertebrae, flip the bird over and firmly press down on the breast to crack the bone so the bird lays flat.

1. Next salt the chicken liberally with sea salt, get every nook and cranny, if you're looking for a measurement, think in the area of 3-4 tsp.

2. Place your chicken in a snug container of the baking dish, now slather it with dressing. Cover, marinate up to 48 hours.

3. When ready to roast, preheat oven to 375F. Lay chicken breast side up on a sheet pan or baking dish.

4. Drizzle with a little olive oil. Roast for 1 hour to 1 hour + 15 minutes.

5. Remove from oven, let rest for a few minutes before cutting apart.

6. In the meantime, chop romaine, drizzle with olive oil and crumble parmesan crisps over it.

7 . To section off your chicken cut the leg quarters off, these
will come apart with ease.

Next, firmly press down with a sharp knife between the breasts
to separate. Serve!

9. CHEESY, LOW CARB STUFFED MUSHROOMS WITH BACON RECIPE

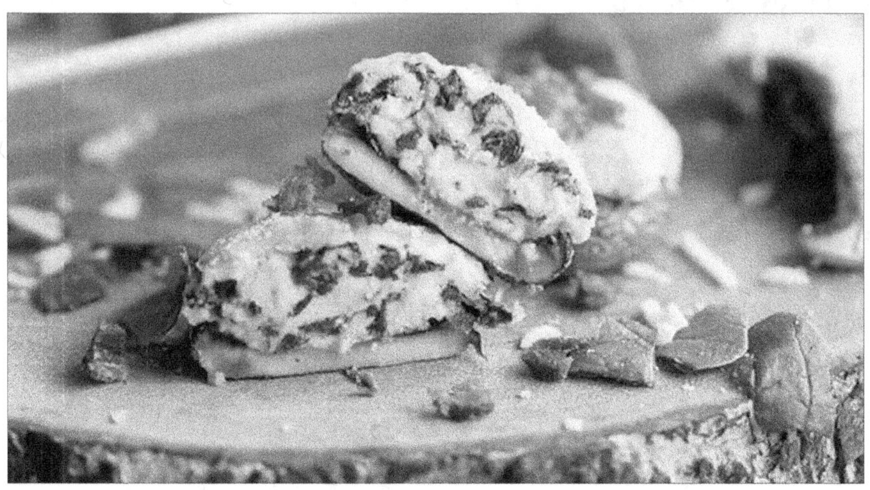

Prep Time: 5 mins Cook Time: 20 mins Total Time: 25 mins

Servings: 14

Ingredients

- 4 thick slices bacon

- 3oz spinach (frozen, thawed, and drained)

- 1 garlic clove (finely chopped)

- 4oz cream cheese

- large whole egg

- tablespoons coconut flour

- 1 cup mozzarella cheese

- 3/4 teaspoons salt

- 1/4 teaspoon pepper

- 16oz baby Bella mushrooms (stems removed, washed, and dried well)

Directions:

1 . Preheat oven to 350 degrees.

2 . Add bacon to a pan and cook until browned and crispy. Remove from pan and crumble into small pieces. Reserve fat.

3 . Add cooled bacon fat and all ingredients except mushrooms and bacon to a large bowl. Mix well until smooth. Stir in 3/4 of the crumbled bacon.

4 . Fill each mushroom cap with the mixture and place in a shallow baking dish. Sprinkle the extra crumbled bacon on top.

5 . Bake 18-20 minutes until golden brown and bubbly.

10. KETO JALAPENO POPPERS RECIPE

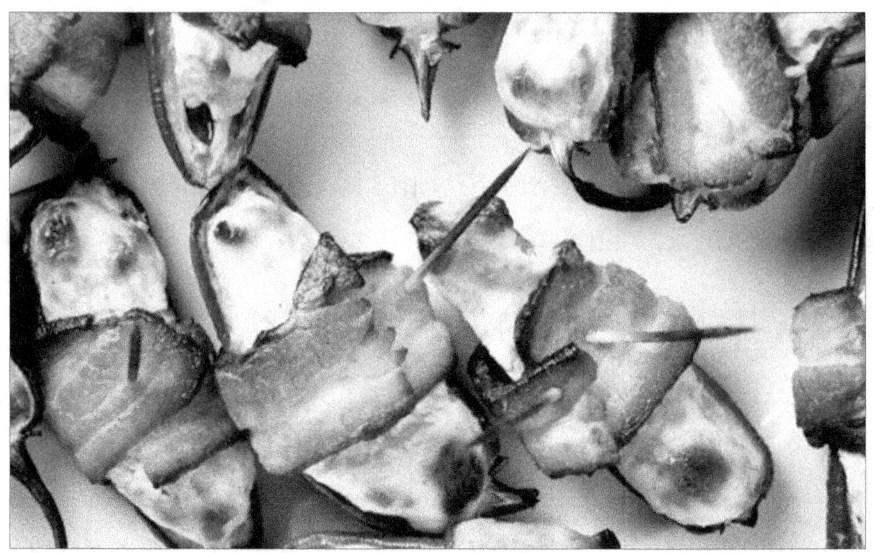

Prep Time: 10 mins Total Time: 30 mins

Servings: 16

Ingredients

- 8 oz cream cheese

- 1/2 cup shredded sharp cheddar

- 1 tsp pink Himalayan salt

- 1/2 tsp black pepper

- 8 jalapenos, halved, de-seeded

- 8 slices of bacon, cut in half

Directions:

1. Preheat oven to 375 degrees and line baking sheet with parchment paper.

2. Place bacon slices on paper towel-lined plate and microwave for 3 minutes. Set aside to slightly cool.

3. In a medium bowl, add cream cheese, shredded sharp cheddar, salt, and pepper and microwave for 15 seconds. Stir together.

4. Carefully scoop cream cheese mixture into a plastic baggie. With scissors, snip off the corner of baggie and pipe contents into jalapenos.

5. Wrap bacon slices around jalapenos and pin with a toothpick.

6. Place jalapenos on a prepared baking sheet and bake for 15 minutes.

7. Increase oven heat to broil and broil for 2-3 minutes, watching to ensure cream cheese does not burn.

8. Remove from oven and allow to cool slightly before eating.

HIGH FAT RECIPES

1. PALEO BACON SHEPHERD'S PIE RECIPE

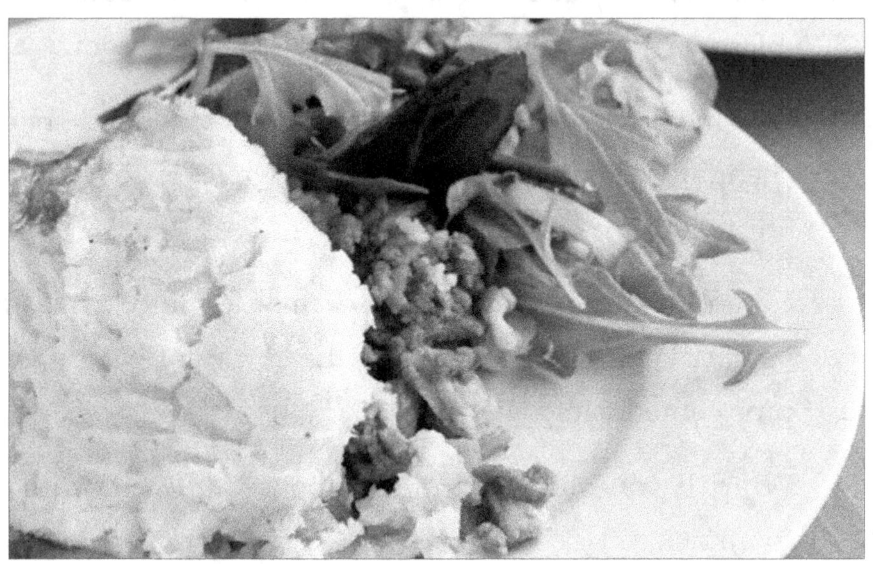

Prep Time: 30 mins

Servings: 16

Ingredients

- Beef Layer

- 375 grams (approximately 15 strips) smoked ham bacon

- 0.75kg (1.6lbs) extra-lean ground beef 2 cups diced carrots

- cup (approximately 2 small) diced onion

- 1 cup (approximately 3 sticks/ribs) diced celery

- cup gluten-free chicken broth

- tablespoons arrowroot starch or tapioca starch

- teaspoons no-salt seasoning

- teaspoon smoked paprika

- ½ teaspoon of sea salt

- ½ teaspoon ground pepper

- Mashed Cauliflower Topping

- heads of cauliflower, florets removed from stem

- 1 tablespoon coconut oil

- 1 teaspoon garlic powder

- ¼ teaspoon ground pepper

- ¼ teaspoon onion salt

- 1 egg white

Directions:

1. Preheat oven for 350F and set aside a 9×13 casserole dish.

2. Add bacon and beef to a large pot and cook on medium-high until beef is no longer pink.

3. Add carrots, onion, and celery. Cook for 10 minutes, stirring every couple of minutes.

4. Add chicken broth, starch, no-salt seasoning, smoked paprika, salt, and pepper. Stir to coat and continue to cook for 3 minutes, until thickened.

5. Transfer to the prepared casserole dish and flatten out with the back of a spatula.

6. Meanwhile, add water to a large pot. Cover and bring to a boil.

7. Add cauliflower florets and boil for 20 minutes, until softened.

8. Drain the water, transfer the cauliflower back to the pot, and mash with a potato masher. Add coconut oil, garlic powder, pepper and onion salt. Mash until super smooth and amazing.

9. Top the meat layer with the mashed cauliflower and spread evenly. Top with egg white and, using the prongs of a fork, fluff up the top, incorporating the egg white to each bit of the top of the casserole.

10. Bake in preheated oven for 45 minutes OR cover and allow to sit in the fridge for up to 24 hours until you're ready to bake.

2. 4-INGREDIENT MAPLE SALMON RECIPE

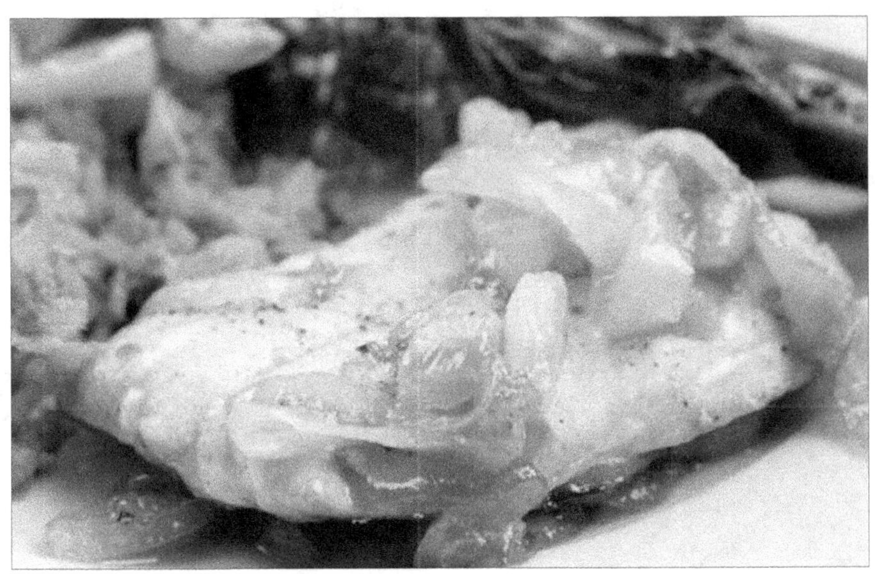

Prep Time: 5

Servings: 6

<u>Ingredients</u>

- 1 tablespoon coconut oil

- onion, sliced thinly

- tablespoons maple syrup

- 6 salmon steaks (approximately 100 grams each) salt and pepper

Directions:

1. Add coconut oil to a large frying pan and melt on medium heat. Reduce heat to low and add onions. Cover and caramelize for 20 minutes, rotating halfway through.

2. Add maple syrup, coating all of the onions.

3. Add salmon, sprinkle with salt and pepper.

4. Increase heat to medium, cover and cook for 10 minutes, until salmon is cooked through.

5. Serve.

3. HEALTHY CHICKEN POT PIE RECIPE

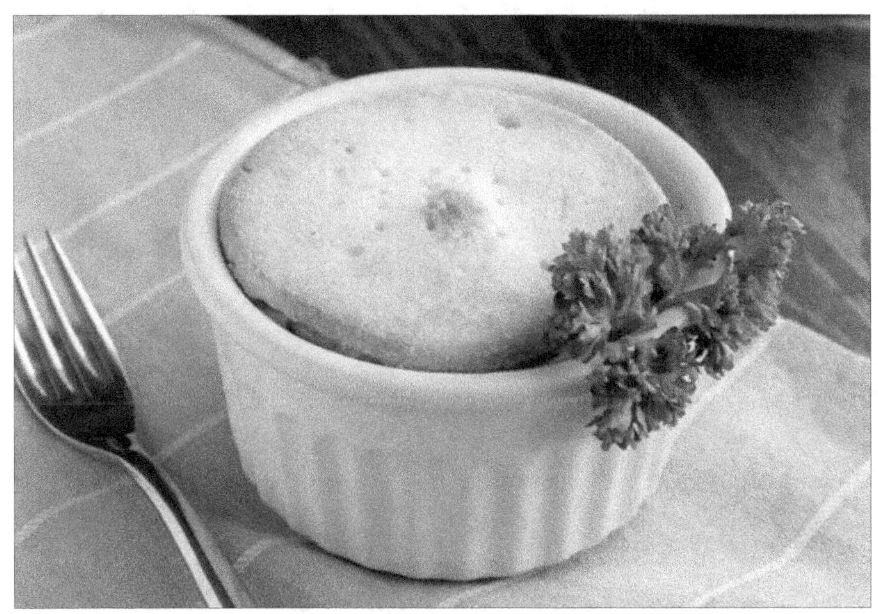

Prep Time: 30 mins

Servings: 6

Ingredients

- 2 teaspoon coconut oil

- 2 garlic cloves, chopped

- 2 small onions, diced 2 ribs celery, diced

- 2 carrots, diced

- 500 grams chicken (approximately 2 half-breasts, 1 whole breast)

- Cream Sauce

- 1 head cauliflower (approximately 3 cups florets)

- 3 cups gluten-free chicken stock

- ½ teaspoon onion salt

- Grain-free Pastry

- 6 tablespoons coconut flour 1 egg

- ¼ cup room-temp coconut oil

- tablespoon hot reserved cauliflower broth

- tablespoons egg white

<u>Directions:</u>

1. Preheat oven to 350F.

2. Add the coconut oil, garlic, onions, celery and carrots to a large frying pan. Saute on medium heat while you cut up the chicken breasts into small, bite-sized pieces.

3. Add chicken to the pan. Cover and cook until no longer pink, about 10 minutes.

4 . Remove the cover and cook for 2 minutes to allow the
juices to boil off. If there are still juices, drain and replace
in pan. Set aside.

5 . Meanwhile, add cauliflower, chicken stock, and onion
salt to a large saucepan. Bring to a boil, reduce heat to
simmer and simmer for 15 minutes, or until cauliflower
is very tender.

6 . Drain the cauliflower, reserving the liquid in a separate
bowl.

7 . Add a cup of the reserved liquid to the jug of your high-
powered blender with drained cauliflower. Blend until
very smooth.

8 . Pour cream sauce over cooked vegetables and meat. Stir
to combine, then transfer to 6 small ramekins.

9 . Meanwhile, prepare the pastry by adding coconut flour,
egg, and coconut oil to your stand mixer, or to a bowl
and mix with a hand mixer.

1 0 . Once mixed well, add hot reserved cauliflower broth.
This will help melt the coconut oil completely.

1 1 . Separate the dough into 6 equal parts. Taking one part
at a time, transfer to a piece of parchment paper, cover
with a second piece of parchment and roll until about ?-
inch thick. Cut a circle out of the rolled dough, I used a

drinking cup. And carefully peel from the parchment, transferring to the tops of the ramekins. Poke the top with the end of a fork. Repeat with remaining dough.

1 2 . When complete, place ramekins on a large baking sheet, brush the egg whites over top and bake in preheated oven for 30 minutes, or until tops are golden and crisp.

4. BEEF KEBABS WITH DAIRY-FREE TZATZIKI RECIPE

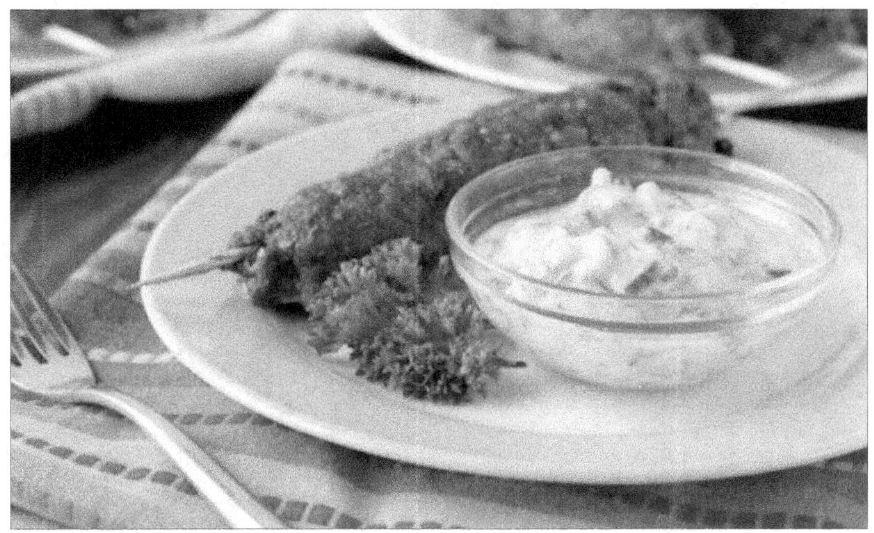

Prep Time: 15

Servings: 6

Ingredients

- Tzatziki

- 1/2 cup mayonnaise (to keep low-carb) or almond yogurt or other dairy-free yogurts

- 1/2 English cucumber, seeded and diced

- 1 tablespoon finely chopped fresh dill

- 1 tablespoon fresh lemon juice

- garlic clove, minced

- teaspoon extra-virgin olive oil

- 1 teaspoon white wine vinegar

- 1/4 teaspoon sea salt

- Freshly ground black pepper, to taste

- Kebabs

- 1-1/2 lb. extra lean ground beef 1/2 small onion, peeled and coarsely grated

- 1/4 cup blanched almond flour

- 1/4 cup dried currants (optional)

- large egg

- cloves garlic, minced

- tablespoon grated fresh ginger

- teaspoon ground cumin

- 1/4 teaspoon ground cinnamon

- 1/4 teaspoon sea salt

<u>**Directions:**</u>

1. Preheat oven to 375F and place 6 bamboo skewers in water.

2. To make the tzatziki, cut the cucumber in half lengthwise and remove seeds with a spoon. Chop up into small pieces.

3. Mince garlic into a bowl with all ingredients. Stir to combine, cover and place in the refrigerator to help develop the flavors while you cook the kebabs.

4. To make the kebabs, drop all ingredients into a large-sized bowl and mix with your hands until incorporated.

5. Separate the meat mixture into 6 even portions and begin to shape handfuls of the meat mixture into sausage-like shapes, about 5 inches long around the soaked skewers.

6. Place completed kebabs on a parchment paper lined baking sheet.

7. Repeat with remaining meat mixture. Once complete, bake in the preheated oven for 2530 minutes or until internal temperature reaches 160F.

8. Remove from the oven, the plate with tzatziki and serve.

5. PALEO QUICHE WITH
A NUT-FREE + GRAIN-FREE CRUST
RECIPE

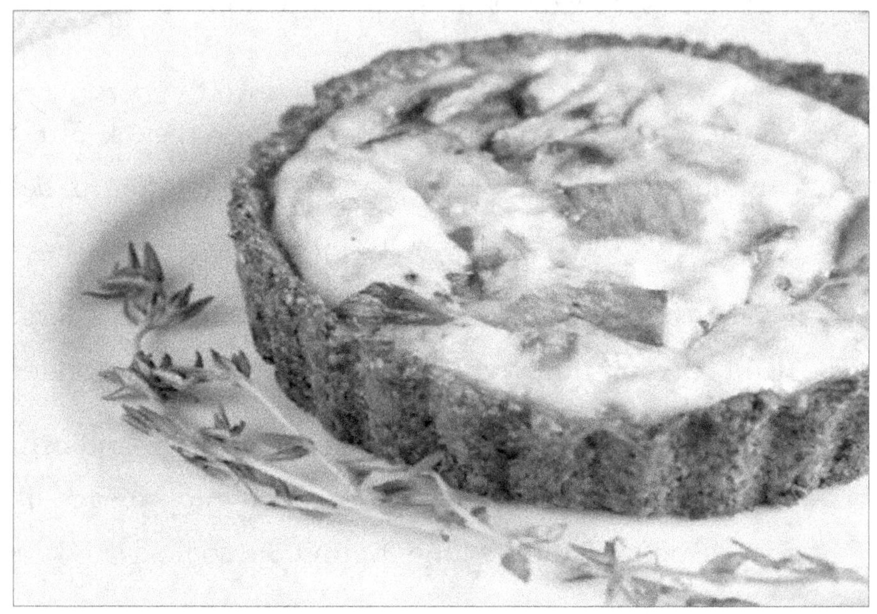

Prep Time: 30

Servings: 6

<u>Ingredients</u>

- Grain-free Crust

- ¾ cup coarsely chopped sweet onion (Vidalia)

- large clove garlic, minced

- tablespoons avocado oil

- 1 teaspoon fresh thyme leaves

- ¼ teaspoon Himalayan rock salt or sea salt

- Freshly ground pepper, to taste

- 1 ¼ cup roughly ground flax seeds or milled flax seeds

- ¼ cup sunflower seeds, ground fine

- Filling

- 1 tablespoon extra-virgin coconut oil

- 1 leek (white and light green parts only), halved and thinly sliced, then well washed

- Coarse salt and ground pepper

- 8 asparagus spears, halved and thinly sliced

- 4 large eggs

- 1 cup full-fat coconut milk pinch ground nutmeg

Directions:

1. Preheat oven to 225F and lightly oil 6, 3-inch tart pans with a dab of coconut oil. Place each on a baking sheet and set aside.

2 . Add onion, garlic, oil, thyme, salt and pepper to the bowl of your food processor. Process until smooth. Add remaining ingredients and process until mixed through. Transfer mixture to each tart pan and mold into the pans, pressing up the edges. Bake for 1 hour and 30 minutes. When finished, remove from the oven and set aside. Adjust oven to 350F.

3 . Meanwhile, heat coconut oil in a medium-sized frying pan on medium heat. Add leek, asparagus, salt, and pepper and saute for 8 to 10 minutes, until golden. Remove from heat and set aside.

4 . Whisk eggs, coconut milk, and nutmeg in a small bowl.

5 . Transfer cooked asparagus mixture to the cooked crust, then pour egg mixture over top. Cook in a 350F oven for 30-35 minutes until tops are lightly brown. Allow sitting for 10 minutes before serving.

6. BEER & BACON CHICKEN
WITH GRAVY RECIPE

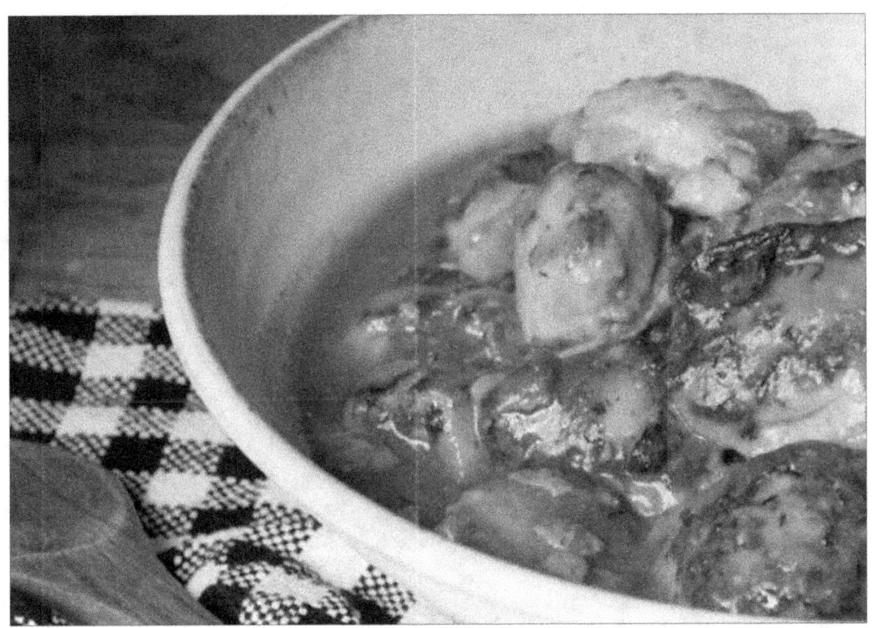

Prep Time: 10 mins

Servings: 6

Ingredients

- 3 tablespoons all-purpose gluten-free flour

- 1 kg (approximately 16) boneless, skinless chicken thighs

- 5 slices beef, pork or turkey bacon, cooked until crispy and crumbled into small pieces

- 12 oz. gluten-free beer (this is my favorite gluten-free beer to cook with)

- ½ cup gluten-free chicken broth

- 2 tablespoons barbecue sauce

- 1 teaspoon dried oregano

- ½ teaspoon dried thyme leaves

- ¼ teaspoon of sea salt

- ¼ teaspoon freshly ground pepper

- tablespoon water

- teaspoons tapioca starch or arrowroot starch

Directions:

1. Place flour in a large bowl and add chicken thighs to it, toss around, until all pieces are coated.

2. Lay the thighs in the bottom of your slow cooker.

3. Combine bacon pieces, beer, broth, barbecue sauce and spices in a medium-sized bowl. Stir to mix. Then, pour over the chicken in the slow cooker.

4. Cover with the lid and cook on Low for 8 to 9 hours or High for 4 to 4-1/2 hours.

5. Once complete, combine water and starch in a small bowl. Set aside.

6. Remove chicken with a slotted spoon and place in a bowl. Cover with foil to keep warm.

7. Stir starch mixture in with leftover chicken liquids. Whisk until combined. Cover and cook, on Low, for 15 minutes.

8. Drizzle the gravy over the chicken and serve.

7. FLAXEED FOCACCLA BREAD RECIPE

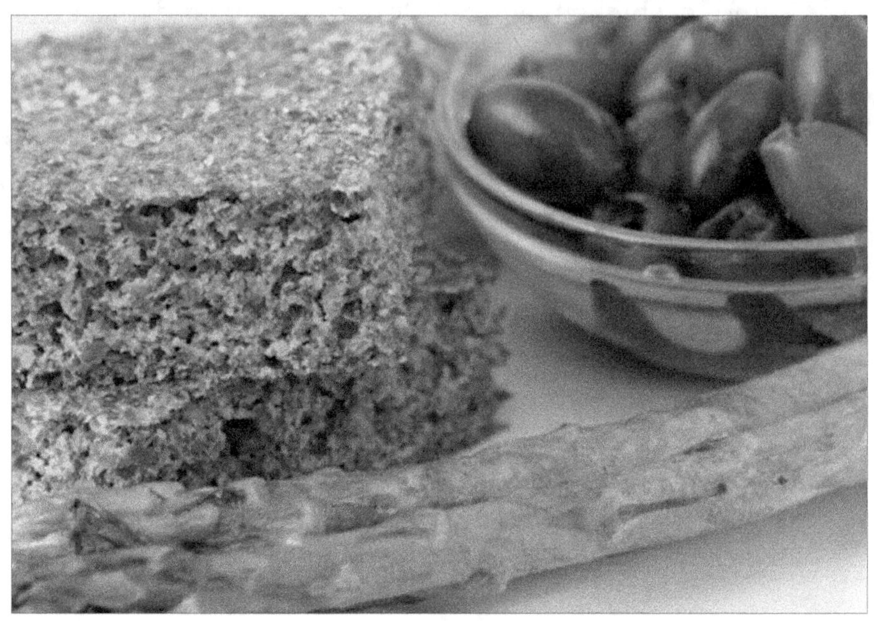

Prep Time: 10 mins

Servings: 12

<u>Ingredients</u>

- 2 cups roughly ground flaxseed

- 1 tablespoon gluten-free baking powder

- 1 tablespoon Italian herb mix

- 1 teaspoon of sea salt

- 5 large eggs

- 1/2 cup water

- 1/3 cup avocado oil or light olive oil

Directions:

1. Preheat oven to 350F and line a 13×9 baking pan with parchment paper draped over the sides. Set asideCombine flaxseed with baking powder, herb mix and sea salt in a large bowl. Whisk to combine fully and set aside.

2. Add eggs, water, and oil to the jug of your high-powered blender. Blend on high for 30 seconds, until foamy.

3. Transfer liquid mixture to the bowl with the flaxseed mixture.

4. Stir with a spatula, just until incorporated. The mixture will be very fluffy. Once incorporated, allow to sit for 3 minutes.

5. Drop mixture into prepared baking pan. Smooth with the back of the spatula and transfer the pan to the preheated oven.

6. Bake bread for 20 minutes, until the top, is golden. Remove from the oven and lift bread (from the parchment paper sides) to a cooling rack. Peel the

parchment paper from the bottom of the bread and allow the bread to cool on the cooling rack for an hour.

7. Cut into 12 pieces.

8. Bread can be toasted or frozen. Keeps in the fridge for 3-4 days and in the freezer for up to 3 months

8. MACADAMIA NUT HUMMUS RECIPE

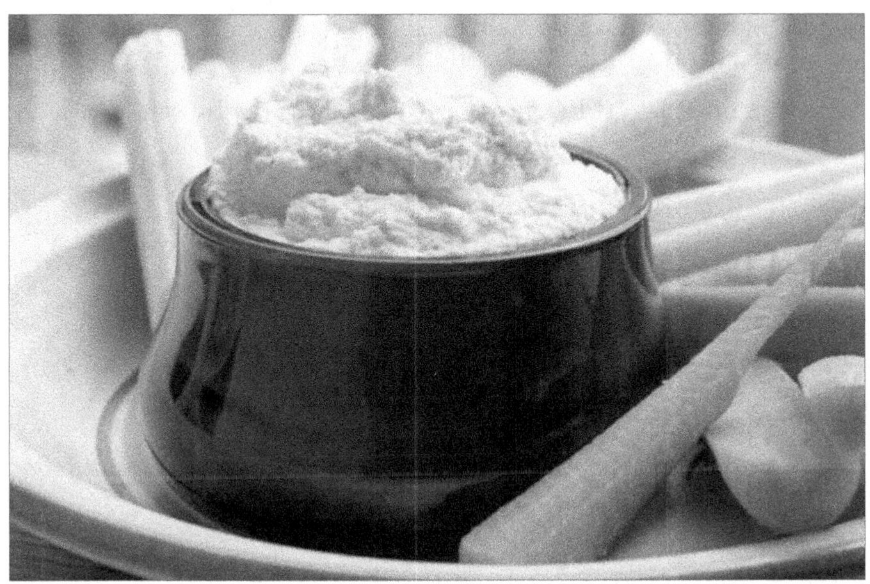

Prep Time: 5

Servings: 8

<u>Ingredients</u>

- 1 cup raw macadamia nuts, soaked in water for 24 hours, drained and rinsed 2-3 cloves garlic

- 3 tablespoons fresh lemon juice

- 2-3 tablespoons water 2 tablespoons tahini pinch cayenne pepper

- sea salt and freshly ground pepper, to taste

Directions:

1. Add all ingredients to the bowl of your food processor or high powered blender and blend on high until smooth.

2. Serve and enjoy.

9.FREE CREAM SAUCE RECIPE-

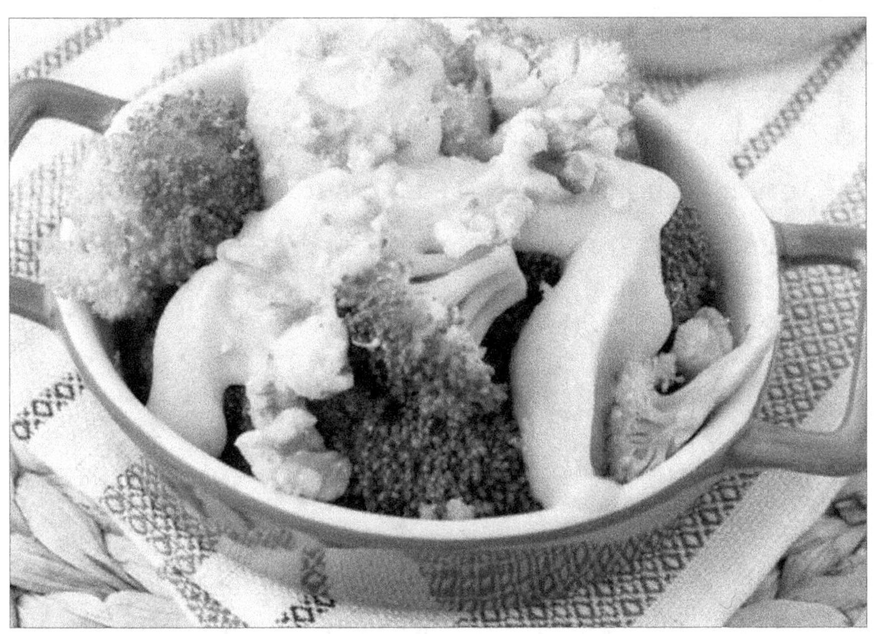

Prep Time: 10 mins

Servings: 8

<u>Ingredients</u>

- 1 large head cauliflower

- 1 clove garlic

- 4 cups homemade broth

- 1 teaspoon onion powder

- 1/2 teaspoon sea salt

- 1/4 teaspoon freshly ground pepper

Directions:

1 . Add cauliflower, garlic, and broth to the pot. Cover and bring to boil. Reduce heat to simmer and cook for 20 minutes.

2 . Drain, reserving the liquid.

3 . Add remaining ingredients with 1/3 cup reserved liquid to your high-powered blender. Blend on high for 30 seconds, until very smooth.

4 . Add to any recipe that calls for creamed soup or drizzle on vegetables, chicken, pulses, grain bowls, whatever!

5 . Can be frozen for up to 3 months. Keeps well in the fridge for 3-4 days.

10. DELECTABLE BACON MAYONNAISE RECIPE

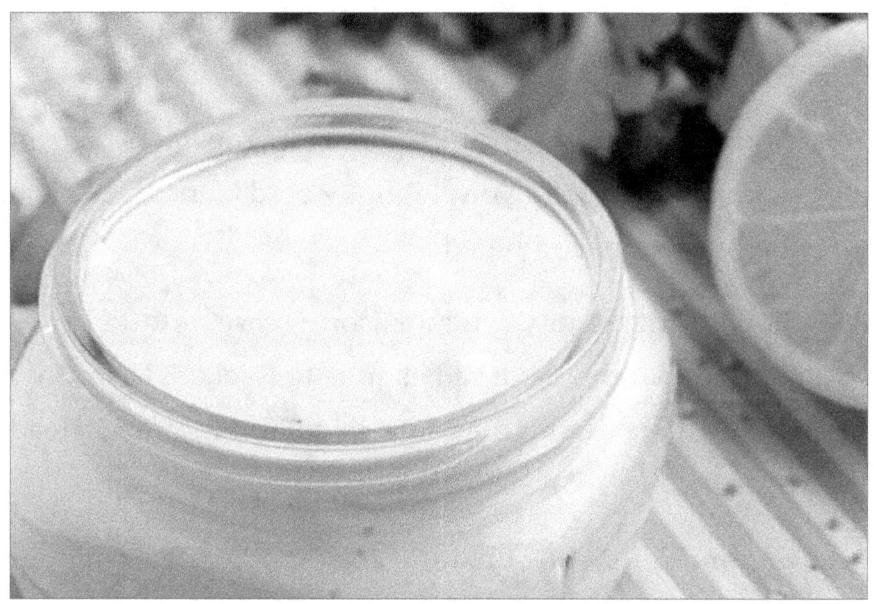

Prep Time: 5 mins

Servings: 10

<u>Ingredients</u>

- 1 egg or 2 egg yolks

- 1 tablespoon fresh lemon juice

- 1 tablespoon white wine vinegar

- 1 teaspoon dijon mustard, optional

- 1/4 teaspoon sea salt or Himalayan rock salt

- Freshly ground pepper, to taste

- 1 cup bacon grease, warmed

Directions:

1. Add the egg, lemon juice, vinegar, mustard, salt and pepper to the jug of your highpowered blender. Blend on medium, until combined.

2. Slowly drizzle in warmed bacon grease, a little bit at a time so that the mixture has time to thicken. Drizzling it should take about 1 minute in total. Slow and steady wins the race!

3. Continue to run mixture for another 1-2 minutes, allowing it to thicken.

4. Transfer to a wide-mouth mason jar, cover and refrigerate. Should keep in the fridge for up to 5 days.

11. NACHO CHEESE CAULIFLOWER TOTS RECIPE

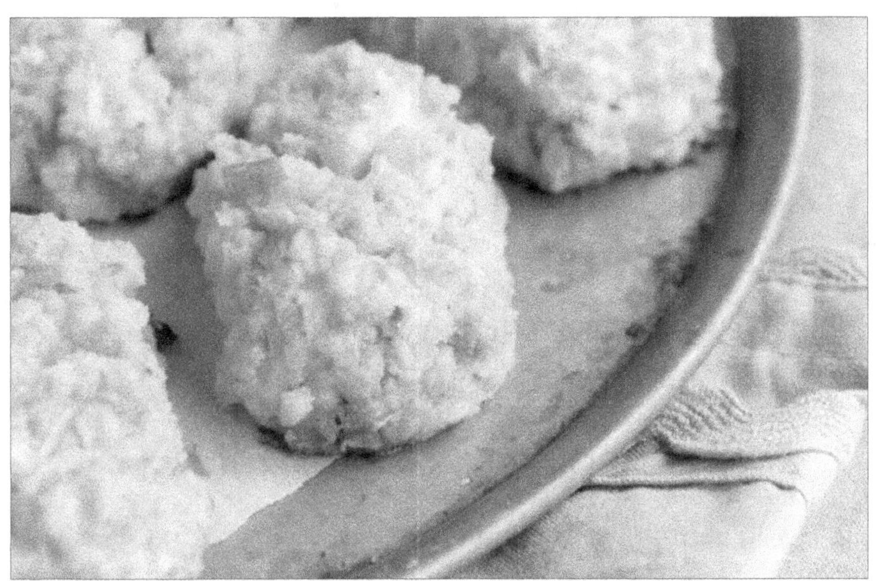

Prep Time: 15 mins

Servings: 16

<u>Ingredients</u>

- 2 cups chopped cauliflower, boiled for 4 minutes, drained & patted dry

- egg

- tablespoon chopped white onion

- 2 tablespoon lemon juice

- 2 teaspoons grapeseed oil ¼ red bell pepper ½ teaspoon liquid aminos

- ½ teaspoon ground cumin

- ½ teaspoon garlic powder

- ½ cup almond flour

- ¼ cup nutritional yeast

Directions:

1. Preheat oven to 400F. And line a baking sheet with parchment paper or a silicone baking sheet. Set aside.

2. Add cauliflower to a large bowl. Set aside.

3. Add remaining ingredients, except nutritional yeast and almond flour, to the jug of your high-powered blender and blend until smooth. Pour over top of the cauliflower. Add almond flour and nutritional yeast and stir until combined.

4. Spoon 1 tablespoon or so of the mixture in your hands and roll into a small oval shape.

5. Place on the prepared baking sheet. Repeat with remaining mixture.

6. Transfer baking sheet to preheated oven and bake for 20-22 minutes.

7. Serve immediately.

12. QUICK & EASY VEGAN CAESAR SALAD RECIPE

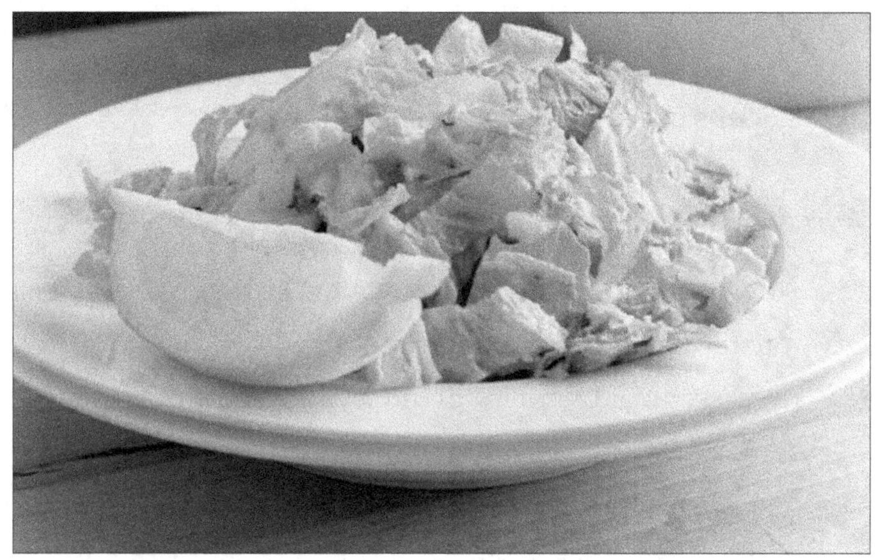

Prep Time: 5 mins

Servings: 4

Ingredients

- 1 ripe avocado

- 3 tablespoons lemon juice 2 tablespoons water

- 3 cloves of garlic, minced

- 1 tablespoon caper brine

- tablespoon capers

- teaspoons Dijon mustard

- Sea salt and fresh ground pepper, to taste

- 1/4 cup hemp seeds

- 12 cups chopped romaine leaves

Directions:

1 . Add avocado, lemon juice, water, garlic, brine, capers, mustard salt, and pepper to the bowl of your food processor or blender. Blend until smooth. If it needs some thinning out (depending on the size of your avocado) you can add a touch more water. The end result will be the consistency of pudding. Keep it this way to maintain ultra creaminess.

2 . Spoon dressing into a bowl and stir in hemp seeds for that 'Parmesan' feel.

3 . Place romaine in a large salad bowl, drop dressing on top and rotate leaves until fully coated.

4 . Serve immediately!

13. 5-MINUTE VAGAN CREAM OF TOMATO SOUP RECIPE

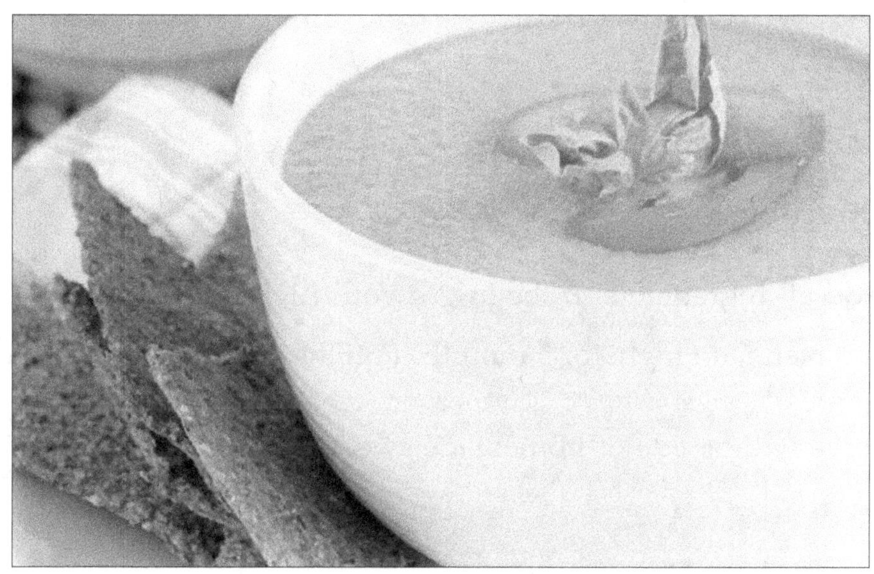

Prep Time: 5 s

Servings: 4

Ingredients

- 4 (375 grams) Roma tomatoes

- ½ cup (85 grams) sun-dried tomatoes

- ½ cup raw macadamia nuts

- 1 teaspoon of sea salt

- ¼ cup (20 grams) fresh basil

- ½ teaspoon white pepper

- ¼ teaspoon black pepper

- 1 clove garlic

- 4 cups hot water

Directions:

Add all ingredients to the jug of your high-powered blender and blend, on high, for 5 minutes until heated through.

Serve with a side of homemade sweet potato tortilla chips, if desired.

14. SWEET ALMOND PATE RECIPE

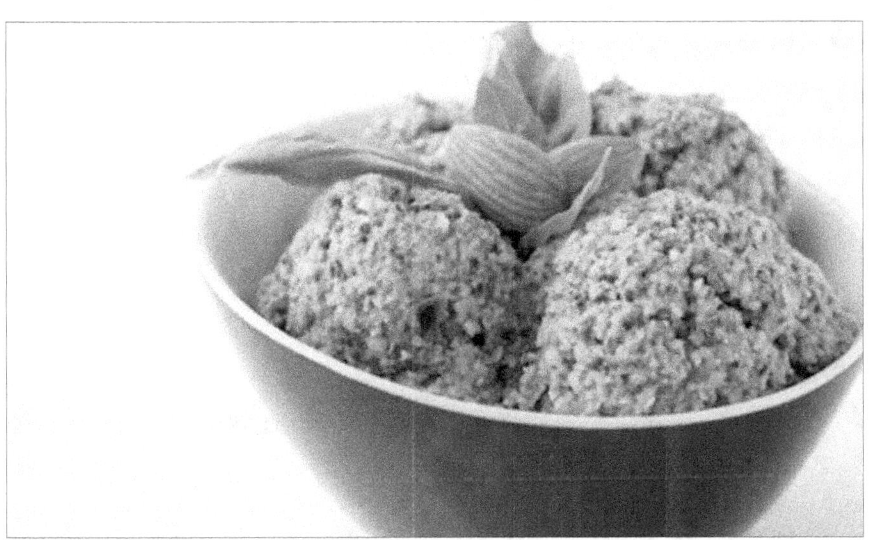

Prep Time: 10

Servings: 16

Ingredients

- 2 cups fresh basil – worked out to be about 3 (40g) packs of basil

- 3/4 cup raw almonds, soaked overnight, drained and rinsed

- 3/4 cup fresh parsley

- 1 garlic clove

- 3 tablespoon extra virgin olive oil

- 2 tablespoon raw apple cider vinegar

- tablespoon lemon juice

- teaspoon raw honey

- 1/4 teaspoon sea salt

Directions:

1. Place all ingredients in the bowl of your processor and pulse with the "S" blade just until chunky. You can either continue processing for a smoother spread; similar to pesto, or stop while there are still chunks of almonds. You can make it a bit chunky.

2. The spread is thick, still relatively chunky, and served best with crackers, a slice of fresh bread, or combined with a simple warm bowl of quinoa and fresh herbs.

15. LOW-CARB ROSEMARY CHIA CROUTONS RECIPE

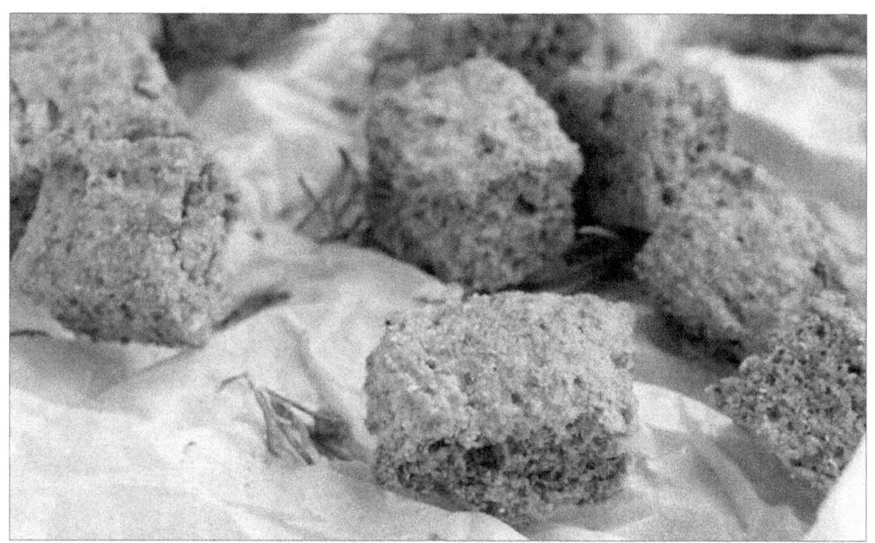

Prep Time: 15

Servings: 8

<u>Ingredients</u>

- 1/2 cup ground chia seeds

- 1/4 cup coconut flour

- 1 tablespoon chopped fresh rosemary

- 1 teaspoon gluten-free baking powder

- 1/4 teaspoon sea salt

- 4 free range, organic eggs

- 1/2 cup extra-virgin olive oil or avocado oil

- Additional olive oil and salt for roasting, if desired

Directions:

1. Preheat oven to 350F and line a baking sheet with parchment paper or a silicone baking mat. Set aside.

2. Combine ground chia seed, flour, rosemary, baking powder and salt in a small dish.

3. Rotate with a spoon until incorporated and set aside.

4. In a larger bowl, combine eggs and oil. Whisk until combined.

5. Transfer dry ingredients to wet, and stir until smooth.

6. Drop the dough onto the prepared baking sheet. Spread to ½-inch thickness. No need for the dough to hit the sides of the pan. Spread evenly with the back of a spatula. Place the sheet in the preheated oven and bake for 20 minutes, or until golden.

7. Remove from the oven and cut into cubes.

8. For crispier croutons, turn off the oven and allow it to cool completely. Remove the parchment paper or baking

mat from the baking sheet and transfer the cubes to the sheet. Place the sheet in the cooled oven overnight. In the morning, coat with additional oil and salt; if desired, then roast in a 350F oven for 15 minutes, until golden.

9. For faster results, once the cubes are cut, remove the parchment paper or baking mat from the sheet, transfer the bread cubes back to the sheet. If desired, coat with additional oil and salt. Transfer the sheet back to the oven and bake for another 30 minutes, until crisp.

10. Remove from the oven and allow croutons to cool completely. Store in a parchment paper bag, on the counter for 2-3 days. The croutons can be frozen, too. To crisp up, toast for a couple of minutes, if needed.

16. THYME AND ONION CRACKERS RECIPE

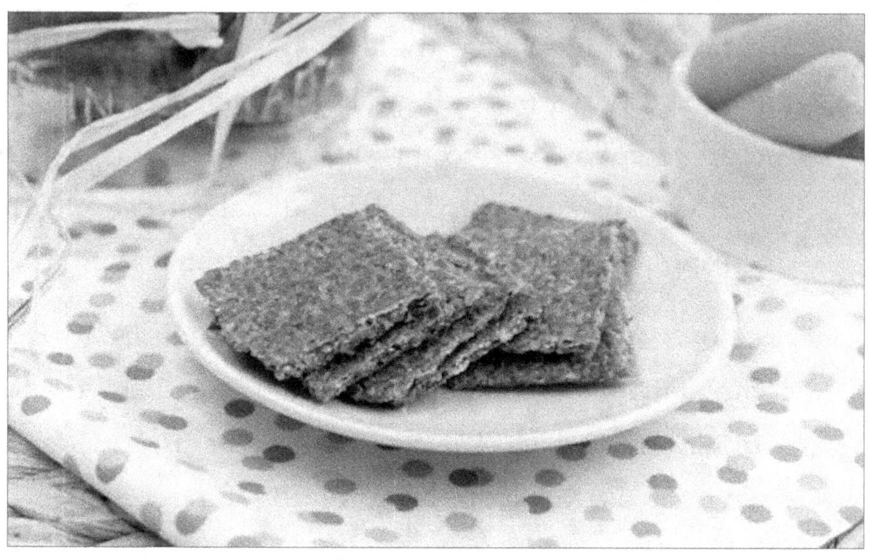

Prep Time: 10 mins

Servings: 15

Ingredients

- 1 cup coarsely chopped sweet onion (Vidalia)

- large clove garlic, minced

- ¼ cup avocado oil

- teaspoons fresh thyme leaves

- ¼ teaspoon Himalayan rock salt or sea salt

- Freshly ground pepper, to taste

- 1½ cups roughly ground flax seeds or milled flax seeds

- ¼ cup sunflower seeds, ground fine

Directions:

1. Preheat oven to 225F and take out two large baking sheets. Set aside.

2. Place onion, garlic, oil, thyme, salt and pepper in the bowl of your food processor. Pulse until onion is completely pureed.

3. Add flax seeds and ground sunflower seeds and pulse just until combined.

4. Transfer to a large bowl.

5. Grab a piece of parchment paper about 10 inches wide. Scoop 1/2 cup of the cracker dough, roll it between your hands to make a ball, then place on one side of the parchment, in the middle.

6. Fold over the parchment (like a book) and then roll the dough between the two pieces of parchment until it's about 1/4-inch thick. Fold away the top half and cut or rip it away. Score the crackers into 1-inch cubes. Keeping

the crackers on their current sheet of parchment, transfer the sheet to a baking sheet and repeat.

7. Bake for 2 hours, flipping halfway through and removing the parchment paper. The baking time will vary greatly on how thick/thin you make the crackers. You want the end result to be crisp, crunchy with no moisture left.

8. Remove from the oven and allow to cool on the baking sheet for 15 minutes.

9. Makes 75 crackers, 5 crackers per serving.

17. PALEO FALAFEL (NO BEANS!) RECIPE

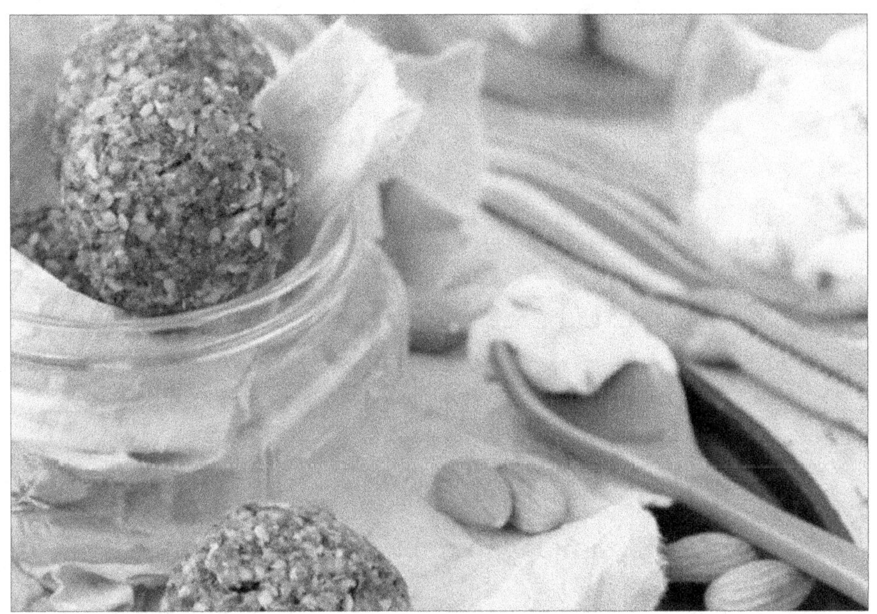

Prep Time: 10 minutes

Servings: 8

<u>Ingredients</u>

- 3 tablespoons sesame seeds

- 1 cup walnuts

- cup almonds

- ½ cup tightly packed fresh cilantro

- ½ cup tightly packed fresh parsley ¼ cup extra-virgin olive oil

- tablespoons lemon juice

- 2 tablespoons dried mint leaves

- 2 teaspoons ground cumin

- 1 teaspoon nutritional yeast

- 1 teaspoon dried oregano leaves

- 1 clove garlic

- ½ teaspoon cayenne pepper

- ½ teaspoon Himalayan rock salt

- ½ teaspoon ground pepper

Directions:

1. Add walnuts, almonds and sesame seeds to a large glass bowl. Fill with water, cover and refrigerate for 12 hours. Once complete, strain and rinse.

2. Add cilantro, parsley, olive oil, lemon juice, mint leaves, cumin, nutritional yeast, oregano, garlic, cayenne pepper, salt, and ground pepper to the bowl of your food processor.

3. Pulse mixture until smooth.

4 . Then add soaked nut and seed mixture. Pulse mixture until nuts is the size of sesame seeds.

5 . Roll the dough; 2 tablespoons at a time, into balls. Press and rotate as you go to allow the mixture to stick. Repeat with remaining dough, creating 16 balls in total.

6 . Place completed balls on food dehydrator racks. Dehydrate at 110F for 10 hours, rotating halfway through. If you do not have a dehydrator, the recipe can be cooked at the lowest temperature your oven will go (180F) for 3 hours, rotating halfway through.

18. GRAIN-FREE GINGER SPICE MUFFIN TOPS RECIPE

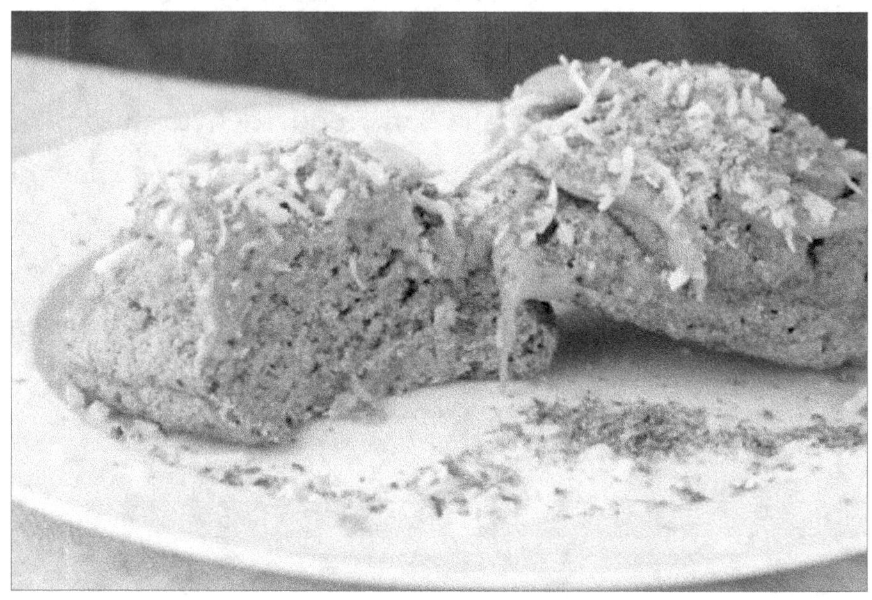

Prep Time: 15 mins

Servings: 4

Ingredients

Wet

- cup egg whites

- 1/4 cup coconut oil, melted

- 1/4 cup lite canned coconut milk

- teaspoon xylitol or 20 drops of liquid stevia

- 1/2 teaspoon pure vanilla extract

- 1/4 teaspoon natural almond extract

Dry

- 1/4 cup coconut flour

- 1 tablespoon freshly ground flax seed

- tablespoon ground cinnamon

- teaspoon ground ginger

- 1 teaspoon gluten-free baking powder

- 1/8 teaspoon ground cloves

- 1/8 teaspoon ground nutmeg

Directions:

1. Preheat oven to 375F and line a baking sheet with parchment paper or a silicone baking mat.

2. Place dry ingredients in a small bowl and whisk until combined. Set aside.

3. In a medium-sized bowl, combine all wet ingredients with a hand mixer.

4 . Add dry to wet and mix until just incorporated, about 20
   seconds.

5 . Let the batter sit for 1-2 minutes to thicken up

6 . Scoop 2 tablespoon piles of the batter using a tablespoon,
   leaving 1 inch between each stack – You can stack each
   tablespoon on top of one another to get really fluffy
   muffin tops. To do so, put a tablespoon of batter down
   on the prepared baking sheet and then put another
   tablespoon directly on top of that one then move on to
   the next pile.

7 . Bake for 18-20 minutes or until a toothpick inserted
   comes out clean and/or the edges are slightly golden.
   Will be absolutely perfect at 19 minutes.

19. 10-MINUTE STRAWBERRY CHIA SEED JAM RECIPE

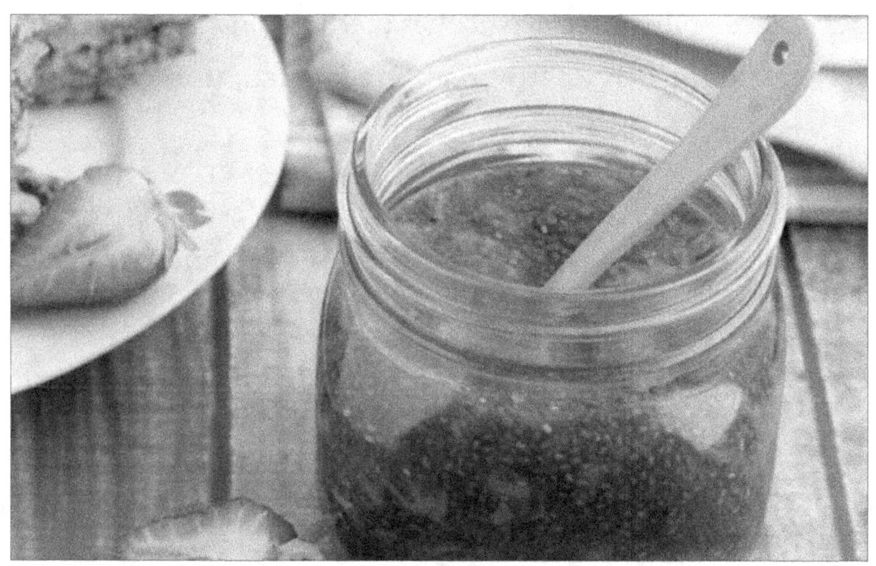

Prep Time: 5 mins

Servings: 8

Ingredients

- 2 cups strawberries, sliced (or any local fruit)

- tablespoon raw, organic honey

- 1/2 cup water

- tablespoons chia seeds

<u>Directions:</u>

1. Add strawberries, honey, and water to a small saucepan. Bring to a boil, uncovered, on medium-high heat.

2. Once boiling, reduce heat to medium and add chia seeds. Continue to lightly boil, uncovered, for 5 minutes, stirring every minute or so.

3. Transfer mixture to a jar and allow the jam to cool on the counter. Use right away or cover and refrigerate overnight to thicken completely.

20. 4-INGREDIENT ITTY BITTY STRAWBERRY COCONUT TARTS RECIPE

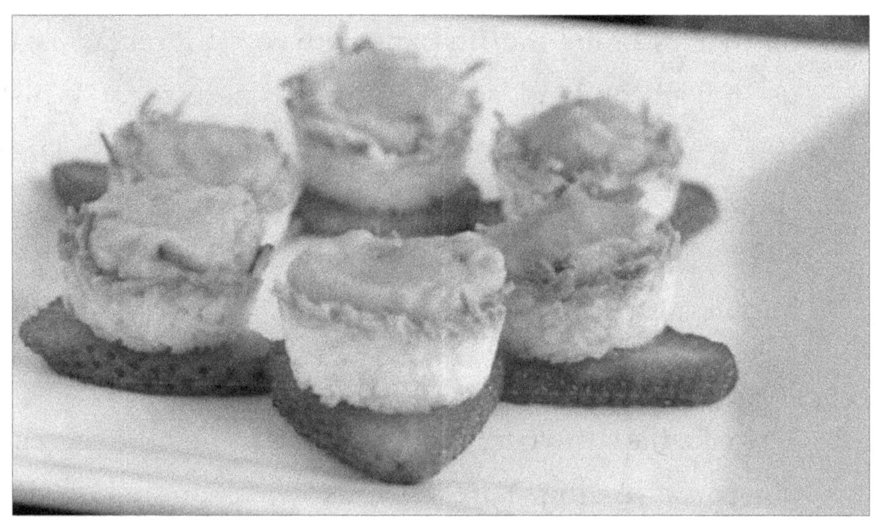

Prep Time: 30 minutes

Servings: 24

Ingredients

- Coconut Tart Shells

- 2 egg whites

- 2 cup of shredded coconut

- Strawberry Coconut Cream

- 4 fresh strawberries, blended

- 1/2 cup coconut butter, melted

Directions:

1. To make the coconut tart shells: Preheat oven to 350F and oil two – 12 mini muffin pans with coconut oil (You can use the silicon kind, so no oiling was necessary). Whisk egg whites lightly and stir in coconut. Drop a large spoonful of coconut mixture into each cup, pushing it evenly into the bottom and up the sides. Bake for 8-10 minutes, or until golden brown. Let cool in the muffin pan.

2. To make the strawberry coconut cream: Melt the coconut butter by placing it in the microwave or soaking the coconut butter jar in a hot water bath until butter is melted. Place coconut butter in a small bowl and mix in strawberries (it will seize up a little bit, just keep warm). Drop into cooled shells by the teaspoon and allow to set in the fridge.

3. Remove cold tarts from the muffin pans and serve.

21. SUGAR-FREE VANILLA BEAN ICE CREAM RECIPE

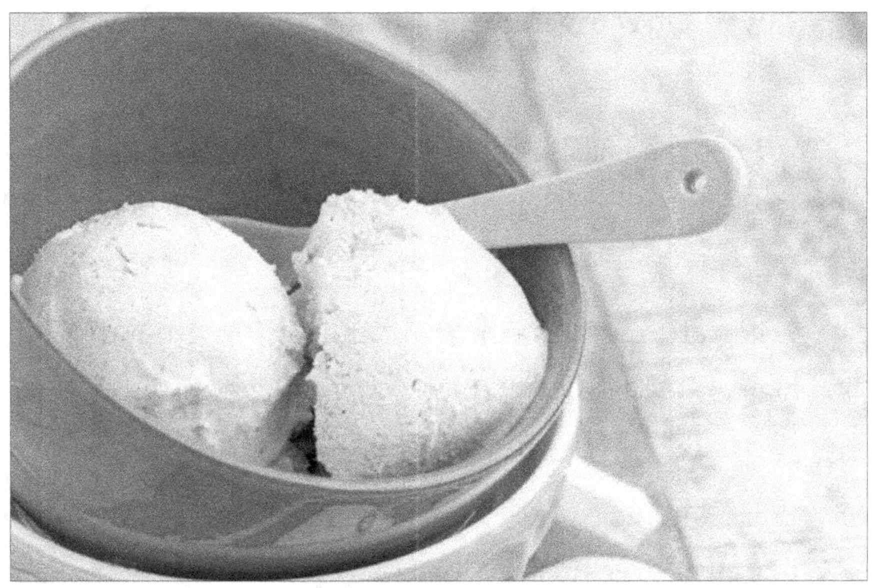

Prep Time: 15 mins

Servings: 5

Ingredients

- 1 cup raw, unsalted cashews

- 1 cup of water

- 1 teaspoon pure vanilla extract

- 1/2 teaspoon vanilla bean powder, optional

<u>**Directions:**</u>

1. Add cashews to a clean glass container. Cover with water; not the water listed in the recipe.

2. Cover and refrigerate for 4 hours. Once complete, strain and rinse.

3. Add soaked cashews, 1 of cup water and vanilla extract to the jug of your high-powered blender. Blend on high until smooth.

4. Transfer to a glass container and add in ground vanilla bean, if using. Cover, shake and refrigerate overnight or freeze for 1 hour.

5. Pour mixture into ice cream maker and follow manufacturers instructions.

6. Consume immediately. Or transfer to a chilled container and freeze for 2 hours for harder scoops. If using in ice cream sandwiches, freeze for 2 hours and sandwich between these Vegan Chocolate Cake Donuts.

22. VANILLA CREME PUDDING PARFAITS RECIPE

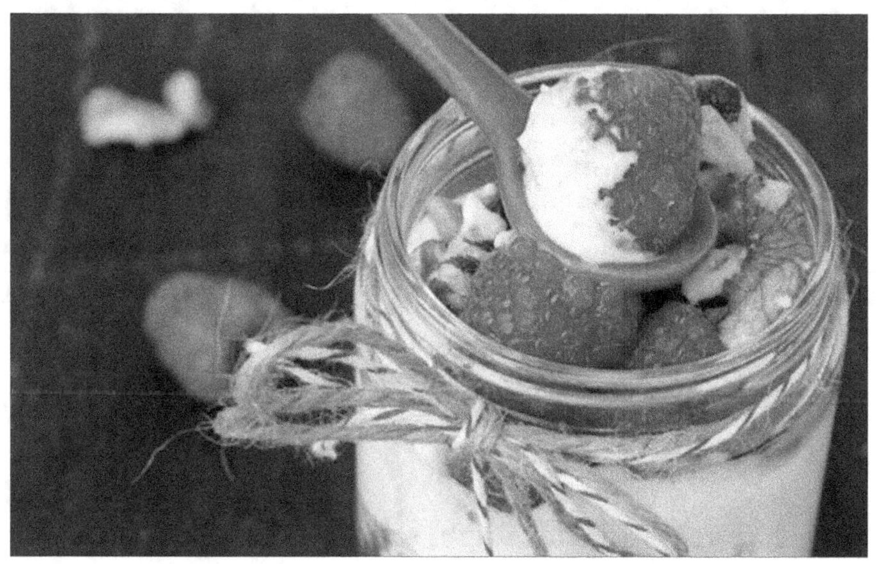

Prep Time: 10 mins

Servings: 4

<u>Ingredients</u>

- 1 can (398mL) full-fat coconut milk, chilled

- 10 drops liquid stevia

- 1 teaspoon pure vanilla extract, alcohol-free preferred

- 170 grams of fresh berries

- 90 grams chopped walnuts

Directions:

1. Add coconut milk, stevia and vanilla extract to the bowl of your stand mixer. Using the whisk attachment, whip for 30 seconds until well combined. Set aside.

2. Mix berries and walnuts in a large bowl. Set aside.

3. Spoon vanilla creme pudding into 4 separate jars, about 3 spoonfuls each. Then, divide half of the walnut mixture between the jars. Spoon a second layer of vanilla creme pudding over top, followed by the remaining walnut mixture.

4. Option to top with a light sprinkle of ground cinnamon. Serve!

23. GRAIN-FREE LEMON COOKIE TARTS RECIPE

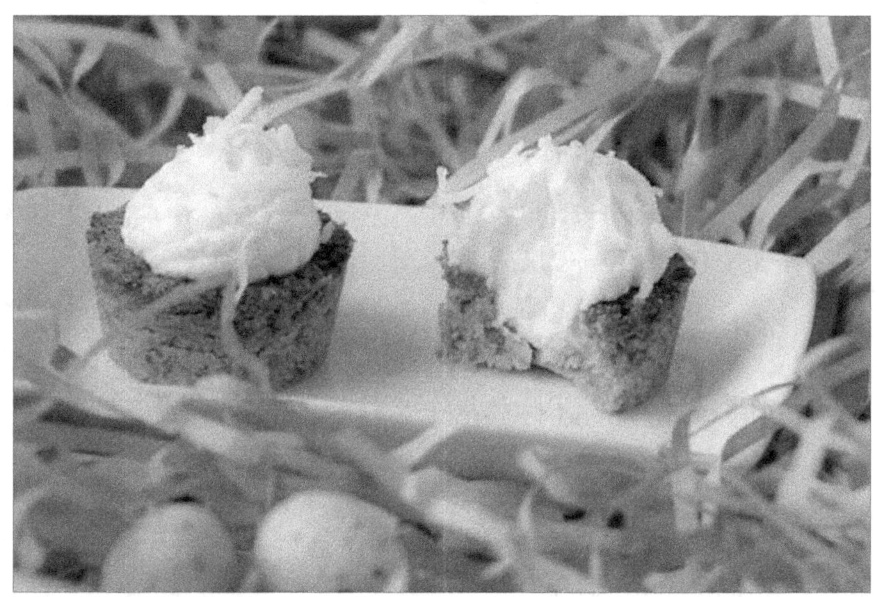

Prep Time: 15 mins

Servings: 24

Ingredients

Cookie Cups

- 2 cup finely ground almond flour

- ¼ cup of coconut sugar

- Zest from 2 lemons

- ¼ teaspoon baking soda

- 1/8 teaspoon sea salt

- ¼ cup of coconut oil

- teaspoon pure vanilla extract

Cream

- 1 can of full-fat coconut milk, chilled overnight and drained of excess liquid

- ½ teaspoon pure vanilla extract

- tablespoon shredded unsweetened coconut

Directions:

1. Preheat oven to 350F.

2. Combine dry ingredients in a small bowl. Then add wet. Stir with a spoon until fully incorporated.

3. Press into 24 mini muffin cups and bake in preheated oven for 12-15 minutes or until lightly golden brown.

4. Using the end of a wooden spoon handle, carefully press into center of each baked cookie to make a 1-inch wide indentation. Cool in the pan for 5 minutes, then gently remove the cups from the pan. Place cups on a cooling rack and allow to cool for 1 hour.

5 . In a medium chilled bowl, beat coconut milk and vanilla.
Beat until frothy, about 2 minutes.

6 . Top each cookie cup with cream, sprinkle with coconut
and serve.

24. GRAIN-FREE BANANA BREAD RECIPE

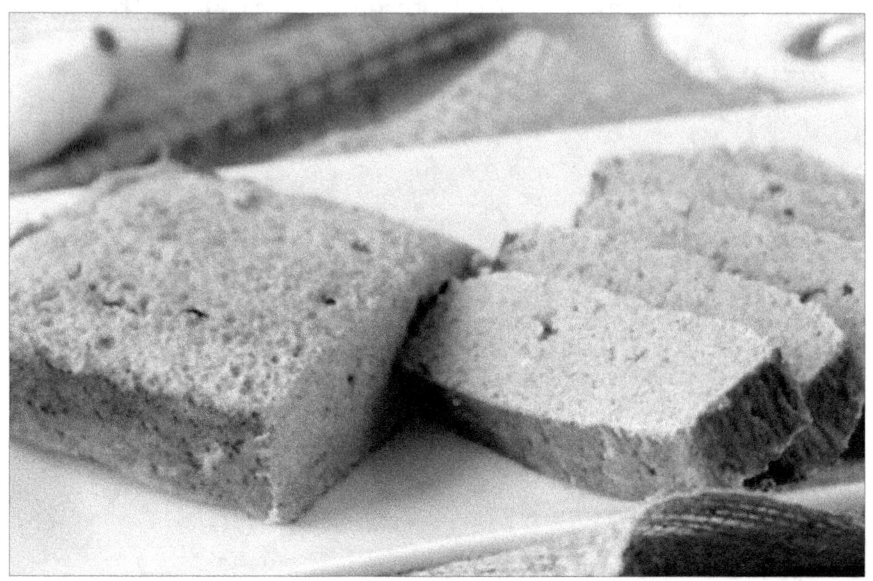

Prep Time: 15 mins

Servings: 12

Ingredients

Wet

- 4 eggs

- ¾ cup mashed banana (2-3 fresh or frozen bananas)

- ¼ cup extra-virgin coconut oil, melted

- ¼ cup non-dairy milk – You can use unsweetened almond milk

- 2 tablespoon unpasteurized honey

- ½ teaspoon gluten-free pure vanilla extract

<u>Dry</u>

- ½ cup coconut flour

- 1 teaspoon ground cinnamon

- ½ teaspoon gluten-free baking soda

<u>Directions:</u>

1. Preheat oven to 350F and line an 8 x 4-inch loaf pan with parchment paper across both sides for easy lifting. Set aside.

2. Combine wet ingredients in a large bowl with a hand or stand mixer.

3. Whisk dry ingredients in a small bowl. Once incorporated, add to the wet mix and mix until smooth.

4. Drop batter into prepared loaf pan and bake in preheated oven for 40-45 minute's or until a toothpick inserted comes out clean.

5 . Remove from the oven and allow to cool for 5 minutes. Remove from pan and allow to cool on a cooling rack for 30-45 minutes before slicing and serving.

6 . Keep stored in the fridge for 3-5 days, or slice and place in the freezer.

KETO BREAD RECIPES
FOR BEGINNERS

1. CINNAMON ALMOND FLOUR BREAD RECIPE

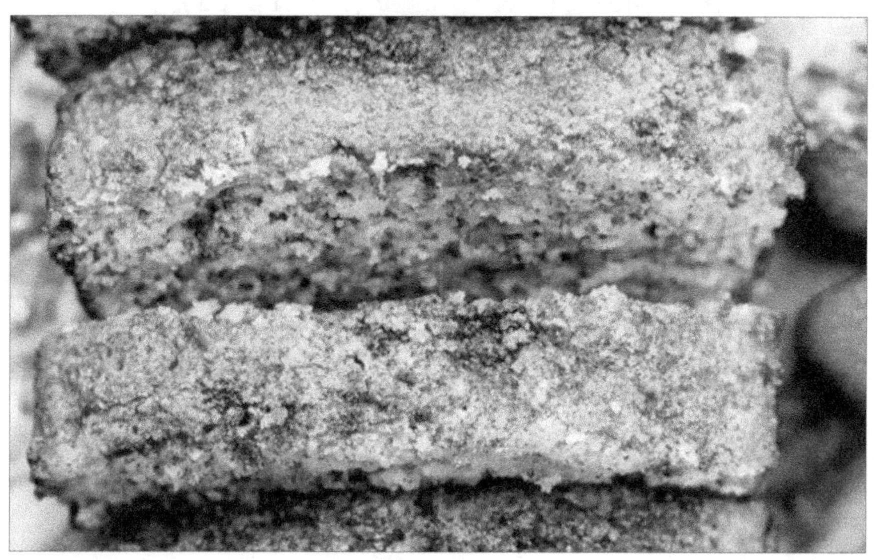

Prep Time: 10 Cook Time: 30 mins Total Time: 40 mins

Servings: 8

Ingredients

- 2 cups fine blanched almond flour

- 2 tbsp coconut flour

- 1/2 tsp sea salt

- 1 tsp baking soda

- 1/4 cup Flax seed meal or chia meal (ground chia or flaxseed)

- 5 Eggs and 1 egg white whisked together

- 1.5 tsp Apple cider vinegar or lemon juice

- 2 tbsp maple syrup or honey

- 2–3 tbsp of clarified butter (melted) or Coconut oil; divided. Vegan butter also works

- 1 tbsp cinnamon plus extra for topping

- Optional chia seed to sprinkle on the top before baking

Directions:

1. Preheat oven to 350F. Line an 8×4 bread pan with parchment paper at the bottom and grease the sides.

2. In a large bowl, mix together your almond flour, coconut flour, salt, baking soda, flaxseed meal or chia meal, and 1/2 tablespoon of cinnamon.

3 . In another small bowl, whisk together your eggs and egg white. Then add in your maple syrup (or honey), apple cider vinegar, and melted butter (1.5 to 2 tbsp).

4 . Mix wet ingredients into dry. Be sure to remove any clumps that might have occurred from the almond flour or coconut flour.

5 . Pour batter into your greased loaf pan.

6 . Bake at 350° for 30-35 minutes, until a toothpick inserted into the center of the loaf comes out clean.

7 . Remove from an oven.

8 . Next, whisk together the other 1 to 2 tbsp of melted butter (or oil) and mix it with 1/2 tbsp of cinnamon. Brush this on top of your cinnamon almond flour bread.

9 . Cool and serve or store for later.

2. LOW CARB GLUTEN FREE CRANBERRY BREAD RECIPE

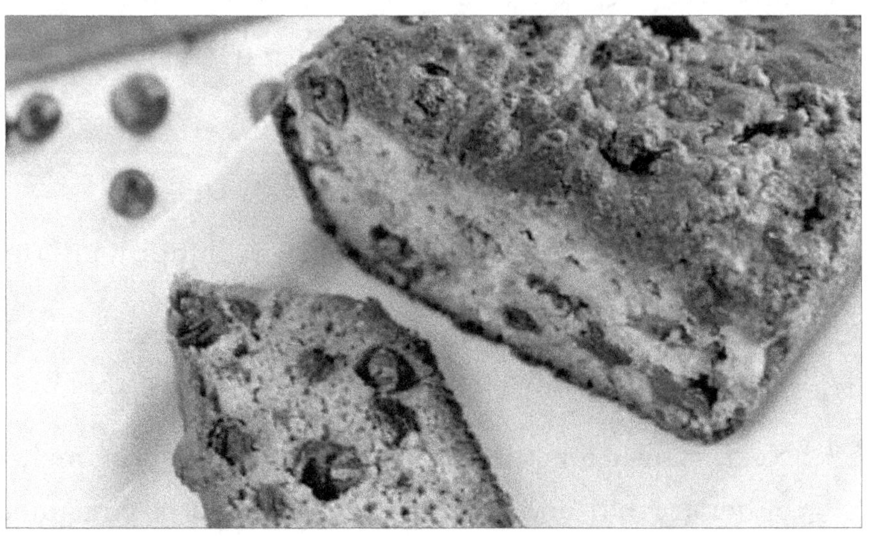

Prep Time: 10 mins Cook Time: 1 hr 15 mins Total Time: 1 hr 25 mins

Servings: 12

Ingredients

- 2 cups almond flour

- 1/2 cup powdered erythritol or Swerve,

- 1/2 teaspoon Steviva stevia powder

- 1 1/2 teaspoons baking powder

- 1/2 teaspoon baking soda

- 1 teaspoon salt

- 4 tablespoons unsalted butter melted (or coconut oil)

- 1 teaspoon blackstrap molasses optional (for brown sugar flavor)

- 4 large eggs at room temperature

- 1/2 cup coconut milk

- 1 bag cranberries 12 ounces

Directions:

1. Preheat oven to 350 degrees; grease a 9-by-5 inch loaf pan and set aside.

2. In a large bowl, whisk together flour, erythritol, stevia, baking powder, baking soda, and salt; set aside.

3. In a medium bowl, combine butter, molasses, eggs, and coconut milk.

4. Mix dry mixture into the wet mixture until well combined.

5. Fold in cranberries. Pour batter into prepared pan.

6. Bake until a toothpick inserted in the center of the loaf comes clean, about 1 hour and 15 minutes.

7. Transfer pan to a wire rack; let the bread cool 15 minutes before removing from pan.

3. PALEO CHOCOLATE ZUCCHINI BREAD RECIPE

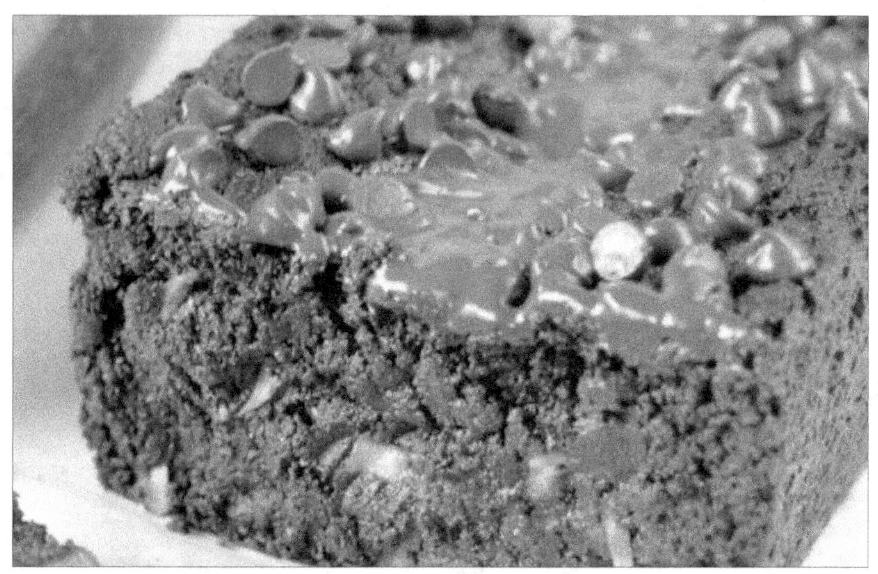

Prep Time: 10 mins Cook Time: 50 mins Total Time: 1 hr

Servings: 12 slices

Ingredients

Dry ingredients

- 1 1/2 cup almond flour (170g)

- 1/4 cup unsweetened cocoa powder (25g)

- 1/2 teaspoon baking soda

- teaspoons ground cinnamon

- 1/4 teaspoon sea salt

- 1/2 cup sugar-free crystal sweetener (Monk fruit or erythritol) (100g) or coconut sugar if refined sugar-free

Wet ingredients

- 1 cup zucchini, finely grated measure packed, discard juice/liquid if there is some - about 2 small zucchini

- 1 large egg

- 1/4 cup + 2 tablespoon canned coconut cream 100ml

- 1/4 cup extra virgin coconut oil, melted, 60ml

- 1 teaspoon vanilla extract

- 1 teaspoon apple cider vinegar

- Filling - optional

- 1/2 cup sugar-free chocolate chips

- 1/2 cup chopped walnuts or nuts you like

Directions:

Preheat oven to 180C (375F). Line a baking loaf pan (9 inches x 5 inches) with parchment paper. Set aside.

Remove both extremities of the zucchinis, keep the skin on.

Finely grate the zucchini using a vegetable grater. Measure the amount needed in a measurement cup. Make sure you press/pack them firmly for a precise measure and to squeeze out any liquid from the grated zucchini. If you do, discard the liquid or keep for another recipe.

In a large mixing bowl, stir all the dry ingredients together: almond flour, unsweetened cocoa powder, sugar-free crystal sweetener, cinnamon, sea salt, and baking soda. Set aside.

Add all the wet ingredients into the dry ingredients: grated zucchini, coconut oil, coconut cream, vanilla, egg, apple cider vinegar.

Stir to combine all the ingredients together.

Stir in the chopped nuts and sugar-free chocolate chips.

Transfer the chocolate bread batter into the prepared loaf pan.

Bake 50 - 55 minutes, you may want to cover the bread loaf with a piece of foil after 40 minutes to avoid the top to darken too much, up to you.

The bread will stay slightly moist in the middle and firm up after fully cool down.

<u>**Cool down**</u>

1 . Cool down 10 minutes in the loaf pan, then cool down on a cooling rack until it reaches room temperature. It can take 4 hours as it is thick bread. Don' slice the bread before it reaches room temperature. If too hot in the center, it will be too soft and fall apart when you slice. For a faster result, cool down 40 minutes at room temperature then pop in the fridge for 1 hour. The fridge will create extra fudgy texture and the bread will be even easier to slice as it firms up.

2 . Store in the fridge up to 4 days in a cake bow or airtight container.

4. LOW CARB BLUEBERRY ENGLISH MUFFIN BREAD LOAF RECIPE

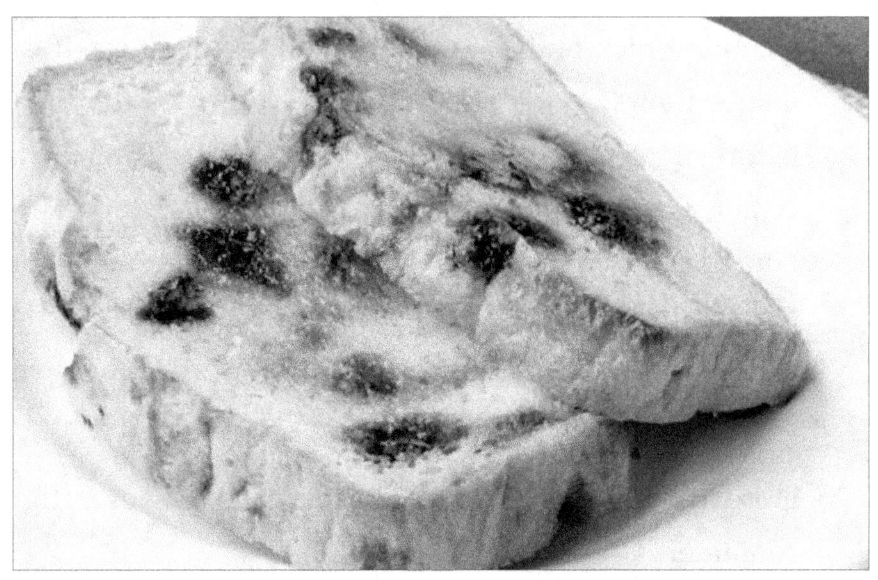

Prep Time: 15 mins Cook Time: 45 mins Total Time: 1 hr

Servings: 12

Ingredients

- 1/2 cup almond butter or cashew or peanut butter

- 1/4 cup butter ghee or coconut oil

- 1/2 cup almond flour

- 1/2 tsp salt

- 2 tsp baking powder

- 1/2 cup almond milk unsweetened

- 5 eggs beaten

- 1/2 cup blueberries

Directions:

1 . Preheat oven to 350 degrees F.

2 . In a microwavable bowl melt nut butter and butter together for 30 seconds, stir until combined well.

3 . In a large bowl, whisk almond flour, salt, and baking powder together. Pour the nut butter mixture into the large bowl and stir to combine.

4 . Whisk the almond milk and eggs together then pour into the bowl and stir well.

5 . Drop in fresh blueberries or break apart frozen blueberries and gently stir into the batter.

6 . Line a loaf pan with parchment paper and lightly grease the parchment paper as well.

7 . Pour the batter into the loaf pan and bake 45 minutes or until a toothpick in center comes out clean.

8 . Cool for about 30 minutes then removes from pan.

9 . Slice and toast each slice before serving.

5. KETO PUMPKIN BREAD RECIPE

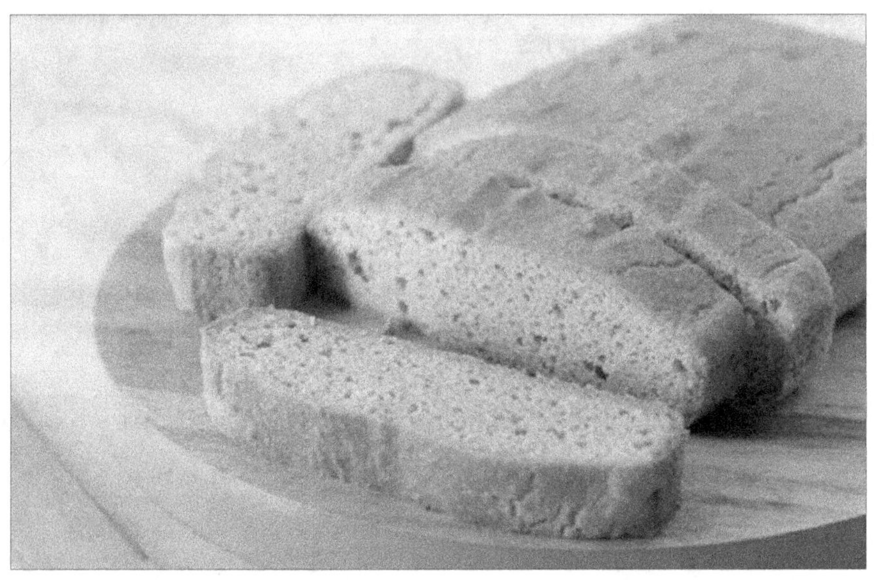

Prep Time: 10 mins Cook Time: 45 mins Total Time: 55 mins

Servings: 10

Ingredients

- 1/2 cup butter, softened

- 2/3 cup erythritol sweetener, like Swerve 4 eggs large

- 3/4 cup pumpkin puree, canned

- 1 tsp vanilla extract

- 1 1/2 cup almond flour

- 1/2 cup coconut flour

- 4 tsp baking powder

- 1 tsp cinnamon

- 1/2 tsp nutmeg

- 1/4 tsp ginger

- 1/8 tsp cloves

- 1/2 tsp salt

Directions:

1. Preheat the oven to 350°F. Grease a 9"x5" loaf pan, and line with parchment paper.

2. In a large mixing bowl, cream the butter and sweetener together until light and fluffy.

3. Add the eggs, one at a time, and mix well to combine.

4. Add the pumpkin puree and vanilla, and mix well to combine.

5. In a separate bowl, stir together the almond flour, coconut flour, baking powder, cinnamon, nutmeg, ginger, cloves, and salt. Break up any lumps of almond flour or coconut flour.

6 . Add the dry ingredients to the wet ingredients, and stir to combine. (Optionally, add up to 1/2 cup of mix-ins, like chopped nuts or chocolate chips.)

7 . Pour the batter into the prepared loaf pan. Bake for 45 - 55 minutes, or until a toothpick inserted into the center of the loaf comes out clean.

8 . If the bread is browning too quickly, you can cover the pan with a piece of aluminum foil.

6. GLUTEN FREE & KETO PIZZA CRUST RECIPE

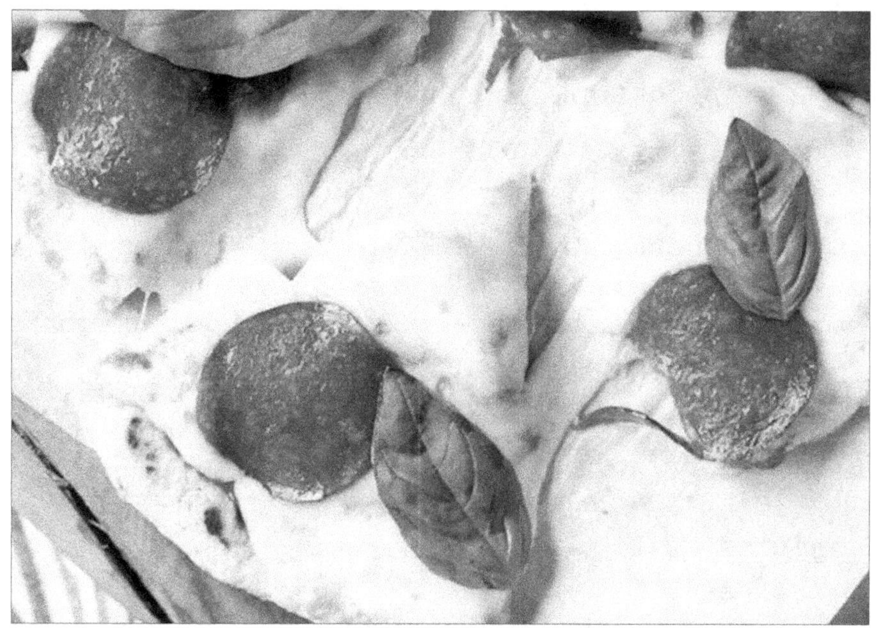

Prep Time: 10 mins Cook Time: 5 mins Total Time: 15 mins

Servings: 10 slices

<u>Ingredients</u>

- For the keto pizza dough:

- 96 g almond flour

- 24 g coconut flour

- 2 teaspoons xanthan gum

- 2 teaspoons baking powder

- 1/4 teaspoon kosher salt depending on whether sweet or savory

- 2 teaspoons apple cider vinegar

- 1 egg lightly beaten

- 5 teaspoons water as needed Topping suggestions:

- our keto marinara sauce mozzarella cheese pepperoni or salami fresh basil

- For the keto dough:

Directions:

1. Add almond flour, coconut flour, xanthan gum, baking powder and salt to the food processor. Pulse until thoroughly combined.

2. Pour in apple cider vinegar with the food processor running. Once it has distributed evenly, pour in the egg. Followed by the water, adding just enough for it to come together into a ball. The dough will be sticky to touch from the xanthan gum, but still sturdy.

3. Wrap dough in plastic wrap and knead it through the plastic for a minute or two. Think of it a bit like a stress

ball. The dough should be smooth and not significantly cracked (a couple here and there are fine). In which case get it back to the food processor and add in more water 1 teaspoon at a time. Allow dough to rest for 10 minutes at room temperature (and up to 5 days in the fridge).

4 . If cooking on the stove top: heat up a skillet or pan over medium/high heat while your dough rests (you want the pan to be very hot!). If using the oven: heat up a pizza stone, skillet or baking tray in the oven at 350°F/180°C. The premise is that you need to blind cook/bake the crust first on both sides without toppings on a very hot surface.

5 . Roll out dough between two sheets of parchment paper with a rolling pin. You can play with thickness here, but we like to roll it out nice and thin (roughly 12 inches in diameter) and fold over the edges (pressing down with wet fingertips).

6 . Cook the pizza crust in your pre-heated skillet or pan, top-side down first, until blistered (about 2 minutes, depending on your skillet and heat). Lower heat to medium/low, flip over your pizza crust, add toppings of choice and cover with a lid. Alternatively, you can always transfer it to your oven on the grill to finish off the pizza.

7 . Serve right away. Alternatively, note that the dough can be kept in the fridge for about 5 days. So you can make individual mini pizzettes throughout the week.

7. KETO BREAKFAST PIZZA RECIPE

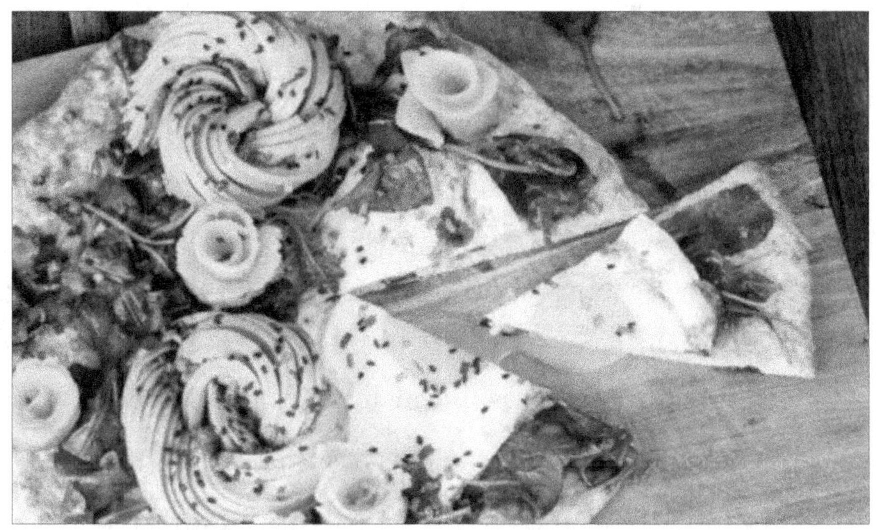

Start to Finish: 25 minutes

Servings: 2

<u>Ingredients:</u>

- 2 cups grated cauliflower

- 2 tablespoons coconut flour

- 1/2 teaspoon salt

- 4 eggs

- 1 tablespoon psyllium husk powder (Use a mold-free brand like this one) Toppings: Smoked Salmon, avocado, herbs, spinach, olive oil

Directions:

1. Preheat the oven to 350 degrees. Line a pizza tray or sheet pan with parchment.

2. In a mixing bowl, add all ingredients except toppings and mix until combined. Set aside for 5 minutes to allow coconut flour and psyllium husk to absorb liquid and thicken up.

3. Carefully pour the breakfast pizza base onto the pan. Use your hands to mold it into a round, even pizza crust.

4. Bake for 15 minutes, or until golden brown and fully cooked.

5. Remove from the oven and top breakfast pizza with your chosen toppings. Serve warm.

8. CRANBERRY JALAPENO "CORNBREAD" MUFFINS RECIPE

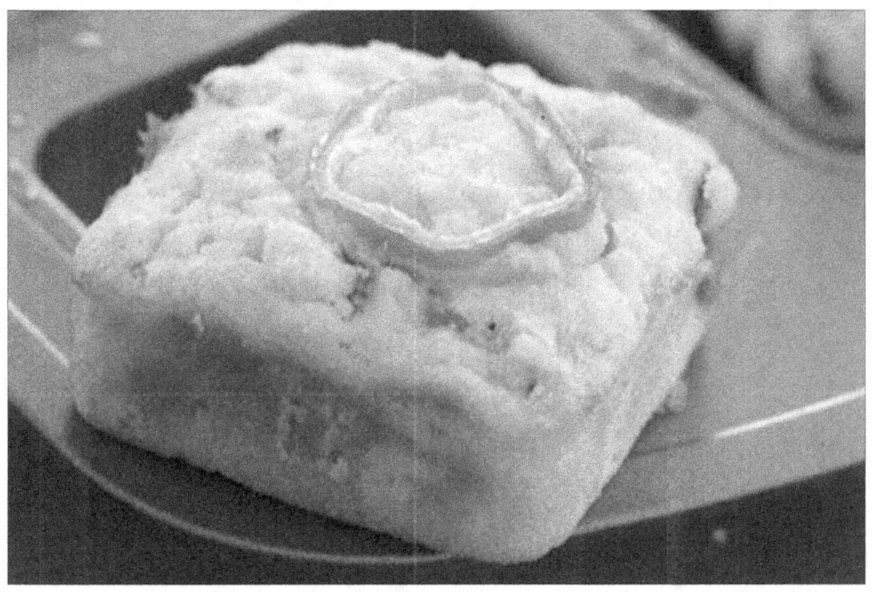

Prep Time: 10 mins Cook Time: 30 mins Total Time: 40 mins

Servings: 12

Ingredients

- 1 cup coconut flour

- 1/3 cup Swerve Sweetener or another erythritol

- 1 tbsp baking powder

- 1/2 tsp salt

- 7 large eggs, lightly beaten

- 1 cup unsweetened almond milk

- 1/2 cup butter, melted OR avocado oil

- 1/2 tsp vanilla

- 1 cup fresh cranberries, cut in half

- 3 tbsp minced jalapeño peppers

- 1 jalapeño, seeds removed, sliced into 12 slices, for garnish

Directions:

1 . Preheat oven to 325F and grease a muffin tin well or line with paper liners.

2 . In a medium bowl, whisk together coconut flour, sweetener, baking powder, and salt. Break up any clumps with the back of a fork.

3 . Stir in eggs, melted butter, and almond milk and stir vigorously. Stir in vanilla extract and continue to stir until mixture is smooth and well combined. Stir in chopped cranberries and jalapeños.

4 . Divide batter evenly among prepared muffin cups and place one slice of jalapeño on top of each.

5. Bake 25 to 30 minute's or until tops are set and a tester inserted in the center comes out clean. Let cool 10 minutes in the pan, then transfer to a wire rack to cool completely.

9. LOW CARB PALEO ALMOND FLOUR BISCUITS RECIPE

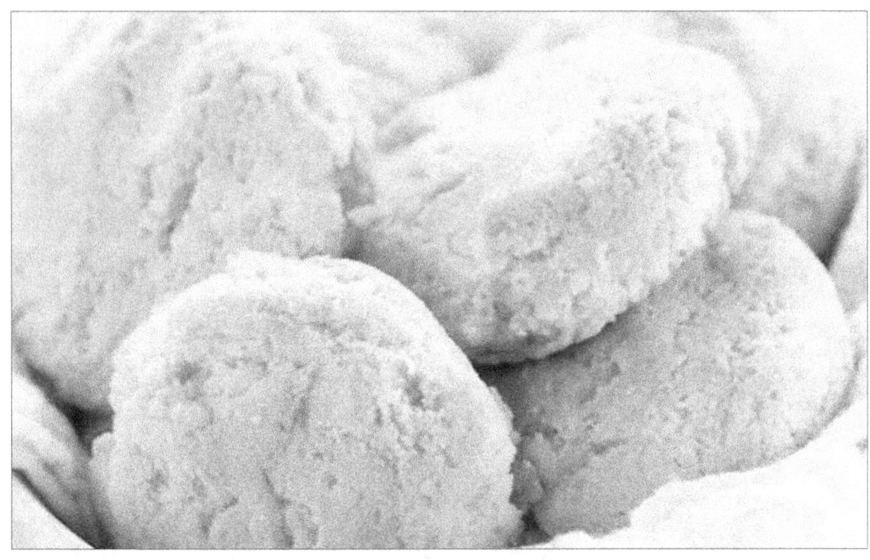

Prep Time: 10 mins Cook Time: 15 mins Total Time: 25 mins

Servings: 4

<u>Ingredients</u>

- 2 cup Blanched almond flour

- 2 tsp Gluten-free baking powder

- 1/2 tsp Sea salt

- 2 large Egg (beaten)

- 1/3 cup Butter (measured solid, then melted; can use ghee or coconut oil for dairy-free)

Directions:

1. Preheat the oven to 350 degrees F (177 degrees C). Line a baking sheet with parchment paper. Mix dry ingredients together in a large bowl. Stir in wet ingredients.

2. Scoop tablespoonfuls of the dough onto the lined baking sheet (a cookie scoop is the fastest way). Form into rounded biscuit shapes (flatten slightly with your fingers).

3. Bake for about 15 minutes, until firm and golden. Cool on the baking sheet.

10. KETO BAGEL RECIPE

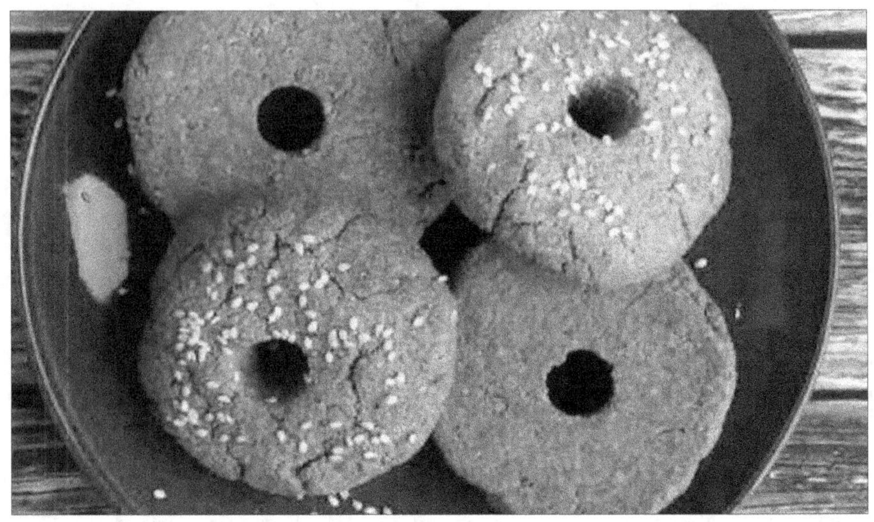

Prep Time: 5 mins Cook Time: 25

Servings: 2

Ingredients

- 1 cup (120 g) of almond flour

- 1/4 cup (28 g) of coconut flour

- 1 Tablespoon (7 g) of psyllium husk powder

- teaspoon (2 g) of baking powder 1 teaspoon (3 g) of garlic powder pinch salt 2 medium eggs (88 g)

- teaspoons (10 ml) of white wine vinegar

- 2 1/2 Tablespoons (38 ml) of ghee, melted

- 1 Tablespoon (15 ml) of olive oil

- 1 teaspoon (5 g) of sesame seeds

Directions:

1. Preheat the oven to 320°F (160°C).

2. Combine the almond flour, coconut flour, psyllium husk powder, baking powder, garlic powder and salt in a bowl.

3. In a separate bowl, whisk the eggs and vinegar together. Slowly drizzle in the melted ghee (which should not be piping hot) and whisk in well.

4. Add the wet mixture to the dry mixture and use a wooden spoon to combine well. Leave to sit for 2-3 minutes.

5. Divide the mixture into 4 equal-sized portions. Using your hands, shape the mixture into a round shape and place onto a tray lined with parchment paper. Use a small spoon or apple corer to make the center hole.

6. Brush the tops with olive oil and scatter over the sesame seeds. Bake in the oven for 2025 minutes until cooked through. Allow cooling slightly before enjoying!

11. PALEO RECIPE

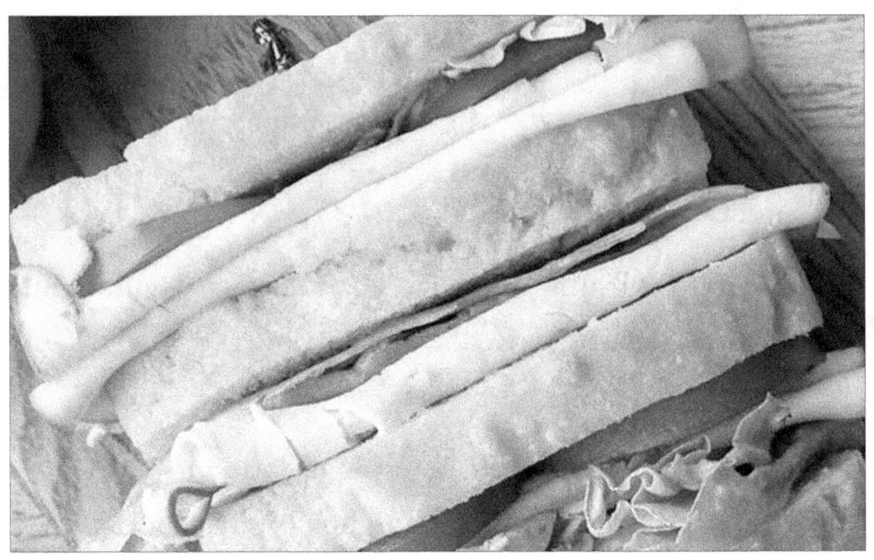

Cook Time: 45 mins Prep Time: 10 mins Total time: 55 mins

Servings: 1 loaf (10-12 slices)

Ingredients

- 7 large eggs

- 1/2 cup melted ghee

- 2 cups almond flour

- 1 t baking powder

- 1/4 t sea salt

<u>**Directions:**</u>

1. Preheat the oven to 350°F and line a loaf pan with parchment paper overlapping the sides.

2. In a large mixing bowl, beat the eggs using a hand mixer on high speed for 1 minute. Add the melted ghee and beat until just incorporated.

3. Reduce the speed to low and gradually add the remaining ingredients until completely mixed and the batter is thick.

4. Pour the batter into the prepared pan and spread with a spatula. Bake for 40-45 minutes, or until lightly golden brown on top.

5. Cool the bread on a cooling rack for 10 minutes before slicing.

12. EASY PALEO KETO BREAD RECIPE

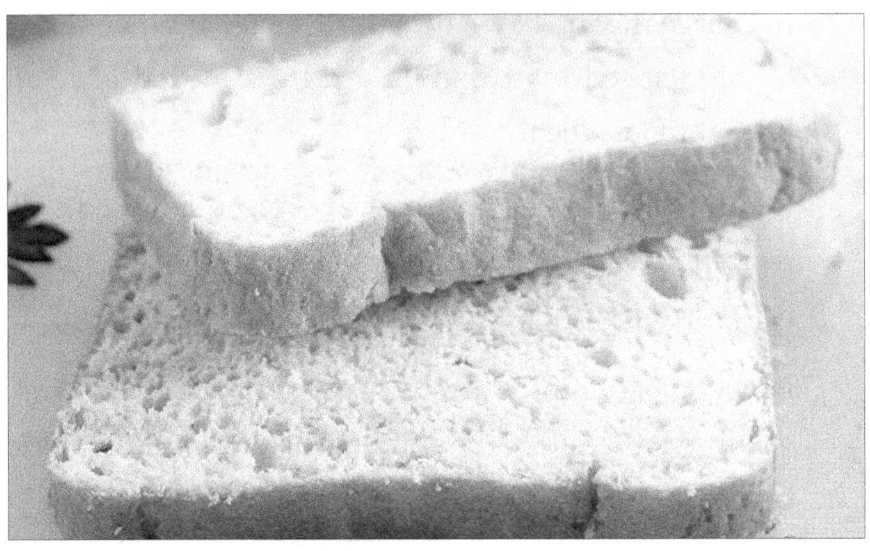

Prep Time: 10 mins Cook Time: 1 hr 10 mins Total Time: 1 hr 20 mins

Servings: 5

<u>Ingredients</u>

- cup Blanched almond flour

- 1/4 cup Coconut Flour

- tsp Gluten-free baking powder

- 1/4 tsp Sea salt

- 1/3 cup Butter (or 5 tbsp + 1 tsp; measured solid, then melted; can use coconut oil for dairy-free)

- 12 large Egg white (1 1/2 cups, at room temperature)

- Optional Ingredients (recommended)

- 1 1/2 tbsp Erythritol (can use any sweetener or omit)

- 1/4 tsp Xanthan gum (for texture - omit for paleo)

- 1/4 tsp Cream of tartar (to more easily whip egg whites)

Directions:

1. Preheat the oven to 325 degrees F (163 degrees C). Line an 8 1/2 x 4 1/2 in (22x11 cm) loaf pan with parchment paper, with extra hanging over the sides for easy removal later.

2. Combine the almond flour, coconut flour, baking powder, erythritol, xanthan gum, and sea salt in a large food processor. Pulse until combined.

3. Add the melted butter. Pulse, scraping down the sides as needed, until crumbly.

4. In a very large bowl, use a hand mixer to beat the egg whites and cream of tartar (if using), until stiff peaks form. Make sure the bowl is large enough because the whites will expand a lot.

5. Add 1/2 of the stiff egg whites to the food processor. Pulse a few times until just combined. Do not over-mix!

6. Carefully transfer the mixture from the food processor into the bowl with the egg whites, and gently fold until no streaks remain. Do not stir. Fold gently to keep the mixture as fluffy as possible.

7. Transfer the batter to the lined loaf pan and smooth the top. Push the batter toward the center a bit to round the top.

8. Bake for about 40 minutes, until the top is golden brown. Tent the top with aluminum foil and bake for another 30-45 minutes, until the top is firm and does not make a squishy sound when pressed. Internal temperature should be 200 degrees. Cool completely before removing from the pan and slicing.

13. MACADAMIA NUT BREAD RECIPE

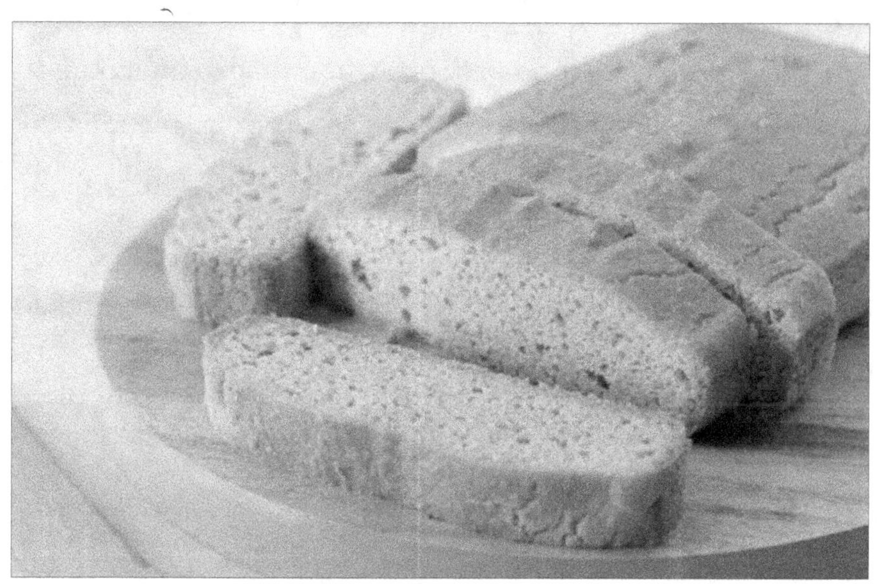

Prep Time: 5 mins Cook Time: 4 mins

Servings: 10 slices

<u>Ingredients</u>

- 5 oz macadamia nuts I used the Royal Hawaiian brand

- 5 large eggs

- 1/4 cup coconut flour (28 g)

- 1/2 teaspoon baking soda

- 1/2 teaspoon apple cider vinegar

<u>Directions:</u>

1 . Preheat oven to 350F.

2 . To a blender or food processor, add macadamia nuts and pulse until it becomes nut butter. If your blender does not do a good job without liquid, add in eggs one at a time until the consistency is that of nut butter.

3 . Scrape down sides of blender or food processor, and add in remaining eggs. Blend until well-incorporated.

4 . Add in coconut flour, baking soda, and apple cider vinegar and pulse until incorporated.

5 . Grease a standard-size bread pan and add in the batter. The smooth surface of batter and place on the bottom rack of the oven for 30-40 minutes, or until the top is golden brown.

6 . Remove from oven and allow to cool in the pan for 15-20 minutes before removing.

7 . Will store in an air-tight container at room temperature for 3-4 days at room temperature, or for one week in the fridge.

14. CAULIFLOWER BREAD RECIPE WITH GARLIC & HERBS RECIPE

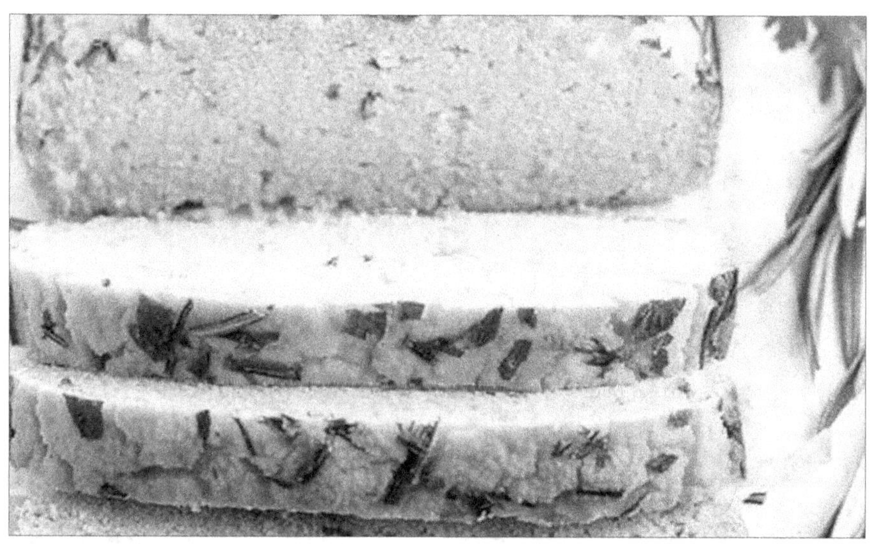

Prep Time: 15 mins Cook Time: 45 mins Total Time: 1 hr

Servings: 10

<u>Ingredients</u>

- 3 cup Cauliflower

- 10 large Egg (separated)

- 1/4 tsp Cream of tartar (optional)

- 1 1/4 cup Coconut Flour

- 1 1/2 tbsp Gluten-free baking powder

- 1 tsp Sea salt

- 6 tbsp Butter (unsalted, measured solid, then melted; can use ghee for dairy-free)

- 6 cloves Garlic (minced)

- 1 tbsp Fresh rosemary (chopped)

- 1 tbsp Fresh parsley (chopped)

Directions:

1. Preheat the oven to 350 degrees F (177 degrees C). Line a 9x5 in (23x13 cm) loaf pan with parchment paper.

2. Steam the riced cauliflower. You can do this in the microwave (cooked for 3-4 minutes, covered in plastic) OR in a steamer basket over water on the stove (line with cheesecloth if the holes in the steamer basket are too big, and steam for a few minutes). Both ways, steam until the cauliflower is soft and tender. Allow the cauliflower to cool enough to handle.

3. Meanwhile, use a hand mixer to beat the egg whites and cream of tartar until stiff peaks form.

4. Place the coconut flour, baking powder, sea salt, egg yolks, melted butter, garlic, and 1/4 of the whipped egg whites in a food processor.

5 . When the cauliflower has cooled enough to handle, wrap it in a kitchen towel and squeeze several times to release as much moisture as possible. (This is important - the end result should be very dry and clump together.) Add the cauliflower to the food processor. Process until well combined. (Mixture will be dense and a little crumbly.)

6 . Add the remaining egg whites to the food processor. Fold in just a little, to make it easier to process. Pulse a few times until just incorporated. (Mixture will be fluffy.) Fold in the chopped parsley and rosemary. (Don't overmix to avoid breaking down the egg whites too much.)

7 . Transfer the batter into the lined baking pan. Smooth the top and round slightly. If desired, you can press more herbs into the top (optional).

8 . Bake for about 45-50 minutes, until the top is golden. Cool completely before removing and slicing.

9 . How To Make Buttered Low Carb Garlic Bread (optional): Top slices generously with butter, minced garlic, fresh parsley, and a little sea salt. Bake in a preheated oven at 450 degrees F (233 degrees C) for about 10 minutes. If you want it more browned, place under the broiler for a couple of minutes.

15. COCONUT FLOUR FLATBREAD RECIPE

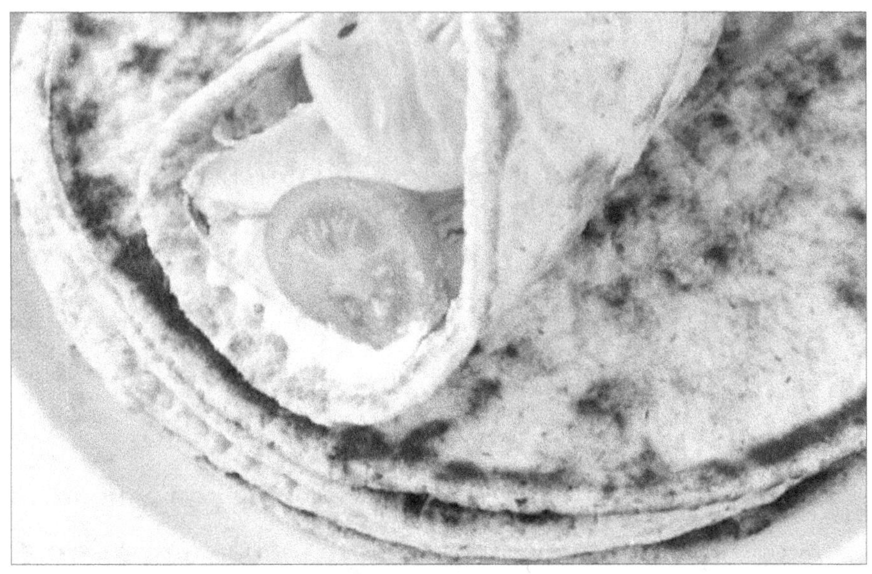

Prep Time: 10 mins Cook Time: 5 mins Total Time: 15 mins

Servings: 6

Ingredients

- 2 tablespoons psyllium husk (9g)

- 1/2 cup coconut flour fine, fresh, no lumps (60g)

- 1 cup lukewarm water (240ml)

- 1 tablespoon olive oil (15ml)

- 1/4 teaspoons baking soda

- 1/4 teaspoons salt - optional

- Cooking

- 1 teaspoon olive oil to rub/oil the non-stick pan

Directions:

1. Make the dough:

2. In a medium mixing bowl, combine the psyllium husk and coconut flour (if lumps are in your flour use a fork to smash them BEFORE measuring the flour, the amount must be precise).

3. Add in the lukewarm water (You can use tap water about 40C/bath temperature), olive oil, and baking soda. Give a good stir with a spatula, then use your hands to knead the dough. Add salt now if you want. I never add the salt in contact with baking soda to avoid deactivating the leaving agent.

4. Knead for 1 minute. The dough is moist and it gets softer and slightly dryer as you go. It should come together easily to form a dough as on my picture. If not, too sticky, add more husk, 1/2 teaspoon at a time, knead for 30 sec and see how it goes. The dough will always be a bit moist but it shouldn't stick to your hands at all. It must come together as a dough.

5 . Set aside 10 minutes in the mixing bowl.

6 . Now the dough must be soft, elastic and hold well together, it is ready to roll.

7 . Roll/ shape the flatbread:

8 . Cut the dough into 4 even pieces, roll each piece into a small ball.

9 . Place one of the dough balls between two pieces of parchment paper, press the ball with your hand palm to stick it well to the paper and start rolling with a rolling pin as thin as you like a slice of bread. My bread is 20 cm diameter (8 inches) and you can make 6 flatbread with this recipe.

10 . Unpeel the first layer of parchment paper from your flatbread. Use a lid to cut out round flatbread. Keep the outside dough to reform a ball and roll more flatbread - that is how you can make 2 extra flatbread from the 4 balls above!

11 . Cook in a non-stick pan:

12 . Warm a nonstick Tefal crepe/ pancake pan under medium/high heat- or use any nonstick pan of your choice, the one you would use for your pancakes.

13 . Add one teaspoon of olive oil or vegetable oil of your choice onto a piece of absorbent paper. Rub the surface

of the pan to make sure it is slightly oiled. Don't leave any drops of oil or the bread will fry!

14. Flip over the flatbread on the hot pan and peel off carefully the last piece of parchment paper.

15. Cook for 2-3 minutes on the first side, flip over using a spatula and cook for 1-2 more minute on the other side.

16. Cool down the flatbread on a plate and use as a sandwich wrap later or enjoy hot as a side dish. You can use a drizzle of olive oil, crushed garlic and herbs before serving! (Optional but delish!)

17. Repeat the rolling, cooking for the next 3 flatbread. Make sure you rub the oiled absorbent paper onto the saucepan each time to avoid the bread to stick to the pan.

18. Store in the pantry in an airtight box or on a plate covered with plastic wrap to keep them soft, for up to 3 days.

19. Rewarm in the same pan or if you want to give them a little crisp rewarm in the hot oven on a baking sheet for 1-2 minutes at 150C.

CONCLUSION

Even though eating bread is often frowned upon when you are on a low carb diet, there are exceptions to this rule of thumb. The key is to get your hands on some easy low carb recipes, as well as low carb bread recipes. If you have these at your disposal, then those delicious buns, delectable muffins, lip-smacking bagels, and scrumptious pancakes, are guaranteed a place in your tummy as part of your low carb diet.

One easy low carb bread recipe is the applesauce muffins, which should be a hit among desperate bread aficionados who have been deprived of their favorite staple. Once you have all the necessary ingredients, and there's quite a lot of it, making it will be an easy and simple process.

It has been noted that usually bread is kept out of the low carb diet, if you wish to add a low carb bread recipe to your low carb recipe book then there are some terrific options for you. There's a variety of range for you in the low carb bread recipes too, you can have muffins, bagels, sticky buns and pancakes too! Well, there are some great bread recipes that you can put on your low carb diet recipe list but make sure you choose the right ones.